Comprehensive Manual of Taping, Wrapping, and Protective Devices

4th ed.

Ken Wright, DA, ATC

Melvin Lewis, PhD, ATC

Scott Barker, MS, ATC

Randy Deere, DA, AT-R

in cooperation with

Cramer Products, Inc
www.cramersportsmed.com

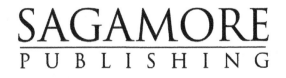

SAGAMORE
PUBLISHING

©2014 Sagamore Publishing LLC
All rights reserved.

Publishers: Joseph J. Bannon and Peter L. Bannon
Director of Sales and Marketing: William A. Anderson
Marketing Coordinator: Emily Wakefield
Director of Development and Production: Susan M. Davis
Technology Manager: Christopher Thompson
Production Coordinator: Amy S. Dagit
Graphic Designer: Julie Schechter
Cover Designer: Reata Strickland

ISBN print edition: 978-1-57167-765-5
ISBN ebook: 978-1-57167- 766-2
LCCN: 2014930902

SAGAMORE
PUBLISHING

1807 N. Federal Dr.
Urbana, IL 61801
www.sagamorepub.com

The authors, along with all contributors to the manual, would like to dedicate this text to all the sports medicine, athletic training, and related health care professionals.

Disclaimer

The procedures in this text are based on current research and recommendations from professionals in sports medicine and related health care professions. The information is intended to supplement, not substitute, recommendations from a qualified physician, qualified health care professional, and medical equipment specialist. Sagamore Publishing, LLC, and the authors disclaim responsibility for any adverse effect or consequences resulting from the misapplication or injudicious use of the material contained in the text. It is also accepted as judicious that the healthcare professionals, sport industry professionals, and students must work under the guidance of a licensed physician, qualified healthcare provider, and medical equipment specialist.

Preface

Being recognized as the comprehensive text in taping and wrapping techniques for healthcare professionals, the fourth edition of *The Comprehensive Manual of Taping, Wrapping, and Protective Devices* has been enhanced by the addition of selected audio and video segments, Kinesio Taping® techniques, and a visual display of protective devices. Obtaining knowledge from recognized experts insport medicine and health care, this text displays and describes a step-by-step process in the application of taping and wrapping products along with a listing of protective devices that could be utilized in preventing injuries. *The Comprehensive Manual of Taping, Wrapping and Protective Devices* features online supplements along with instructor resources.

Online Companion Resources

Online companion resources include videos, images, and other resources the authors have provided as supplemental information for the text. These resources are found online and and accessible only by creating an account using the one-time passcode provided in the back of the text on page 213. For more information about the use of or policies regarding the code for online companion resources, please visit www.sagamorepub.com.

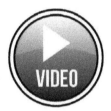 Icon indicates that an instructional video is available for the technique using the Online Companion Resources.

Special Thanks

The authors would like to thank Sagamore Publishing, LLC, Medco Sports Medicine, Kinesio Taping, Johnson & Johnson, and Cramer Products for providing the financial support for this project. Without their support, we would not have been able to complete the 4th edition of *The Comprehensive Manual of Taping, Wrapping, and Protective Devices*. The authors would also like to thank the following individuals for their assistance in the development of this manual: Ms. Reata Strickland as cover designer; Mr. William Tremlett, Mr. Austin Shelnutt, Ms. Kelly Wright, and Ms. Kendra Wright for serving as guest reviewers, and past editors/reviewer (Mr. William Whitehill, Mr. Bud Carperter, Mrs. Katy Curren Casey, Mr. James Dodson, Ms. A. Louise Fincher, Mr. Tim Garl, Ms. Sherry Kimbro, Mr. Donald Lowe, Mr. Henry Lyda, Mr. William McDonald, Mrs. Alice McLaine, Mr. Lindsey McLean, Ms. Lorraine Michel, Mr. Russell Miller, Mr. Ken Murray, Mr. Chris Patrick, Mr. Ralph Reiff, Mr. Ed Ryan, Dr. Patrick Sexton, Dr. Vincent Stilger, Mr. Hunter Smith, Mr. Buddy Taylor, and Mr. Charles Vosler) of the *Comprehensive Manual of Taping and Wrapping Techniques* and *Preventive Techniques: Taping/Wrapping Techniques and Protective Devices* for their input and expertise.

Acknowledgments

The authors are extremely grateful to the following for their meticulous review, comments, and contributions during the development and update of this book:

- E. Lyle Cain, MD, Andrews Sports Medicine & Orthopaedic Center, Birmingham, AL
- George Borden, MSc, AT-R, The Society of Sports Therapists, Glasgow, U.K.
- Samuel Brown, MS, OTC, Southern Crescent Technical College, Griffin, GA
- Rodney Brown, MA, LAT, ATC, The University of Alabama, Tuscaloosa, AL
- R. T. Floyd, EdD, ATC, The University of West Alabama
- Ginger Gilmore, MS, LAT, ATC, The University of Alabama, Tuscaloosa, AL
- Ronnie Harper, EdD, LAT, ATC, Dutchtown High School, Geismar, LA
- Fred Hina, MA, ATC, University of Louisville, Louisville, KY
- Ron Medlin, MS, ATC, Baltimore Ravens, Owings Mills, MD
- Tim Neal, MS, ATC, Syracuse University, Syracuse, NY
- Ron Walker, MA, LAT, ATC, CSCS, The University of Tulsa, Tulsa, OK
- Katherine Wright, PT, DPT, MS, Memorial Hermann Sports Medicine, Houston, TX

Comprehensive Manual of Taping, Wrapping, and Protective Devices, *4th ed.*

Contents

PART I: BASIC FUNDAMENTALS

PART III: KINESIO TAPING METHOD

PART IV: TECHNIQUES FOR UPPER EXTREMITIES

PART V: RECOMMENDATIONS FOR SELECTED PROTECTIVE DEVICES

About the Authors

Ken Wright, DA, ATC

Dr. Ken Wright is a professor and director of the Sport Management Program at The University of Alabama. Dr. Wright received his doctor of arts degree from Middle Tennessee State University (1984), master of science degree from Syracuse University (1976), and bachelor of science degree from Eastern Kentucky University (1974). He has served as head athletic trainer at the University of North Carolina at Charlotte and Morehead State University and assistant athletic trainer at Ohio University. Additionally, he was selected as Outstanding Alumnus at Eastern Kentucky University (2001), and he received the Academic Excellence Award from The University of Alabama. In 2012, Dr. Wright was appointed as a member of the board of directors of the United States Anti-Doping Agency. Since 1990, he has served as a Doping Control Officer during which time he worked three Olympic Games (London, Vancouver, and Salt Lake City). Ken has been involved with the United States Olympic Committee as an athletic trainer, educator, and invited presenter at numerous sports medicine and sport management meetings in China, Japan, United Kingdom, Canada, and the United States. From the National Athletic Trainers' Association, Dr. Wright received the Sayers "Bud" Miller Distinguished Educator of the Year Award (2000), Distinguished Athletic Trainer Award (2006), and Athletic Trainer Service Award (1996). Dr. Wright has numerous publications to his credit, including a series of 13 videos (*Sports Medicine Evaluation* and *Sports Medicine Taping*), a computer-assisted instructional program (*Sports Injuries*), and textbooks (*Basic Athletic Training, Preventive Techniques: Taping/Wrapping Techniques and Protective Devices*, and *The Comprehensive Manual of Taping and Wrapping Techniques*). Additionally, he has served on the editorial board of the *Journal of Athletic Training, Physical Therapy in Sport*, and *Sports Medicine Update*, athletic training education accreditation visits, and various USADA, USOC, and NATA committees.

Melvin Lewis, PhD, ATC

Dr. Melvin Lewis is the National Sales Director for Medco Sports Medicine. He is also an adjunct faculty member of the Sport Management Program at The University of Alabama. Dr. Lewis is a member of the National Athletic Trainers' Association and North American Society for Sport Management. Dr. Lewis received all three of his higher education degrees from The University of Alabama. He earned a doctor of philosophy degree in 2003, master of arts degree in 1996, and a bachelor of science degree in 1994. Dr. Lewis received certificates of training for Carew International Essentials of Branch Management Leadership in 2011, Carew International Dimensions of Professional Selling Facilitator Training in 2010, and The Counselor Salesperson in 2005. He was an assistant athletic trainer for the Buffalo Bills Professional Football Organization for four years. Prior to joining the Buffalo Bills full time in 1996, Dr. Lewis was a summer intern for the Buffalo Bills in 1995 and the Los Angeles Raiders Professional Football Organization in 1994. Dr. Lewis received the SREB Fellowship for Doctoral Scholars in 2000 and the Professional Football Athletic Trainers Minority Scholarship in 1994. Dr. Lewis is a coauthor and has presented scholarly work.

Scott Barker, MS, ATC

Mr. Scott Barker is the head athletic trainer and adjunct faculty for the graduate athletic training education program at California State University, Chico. He received his master of science degree in exercise and sport sciences with a specialization in athletic training from the University of Arizona (1985) and his bachelor of science degree in physical education from the University of Arizona (1984). Barker served for eight years on the National Athletic Trainers Association Education Council Continuing Education Committee and for nine years on the National Athletic Trainers Association Education Multimedia Committee. During this time, Mr. Barker helped with the inception and development of the National Athletic Trainers' Association Virtual Library (online continuing education courses). Barker has received numerous awards in the area of educational multimedia in athletic training including the 2000, 2001, 2002, 2004, 2005, and 2008 National Athletic Trainers' Association, Educational Multimedia Committee, Educational Software Production Contest ATC Commercial Winner; the 2006 National Athletic Trainers' Association, Educational Multimedia Committee, Educational DVD/Video Production Contest ATC Commercial Winner; the 2006 National Athletic Trainers' Association Continuing Education Excellence Award; and the 2007 MERLOT Classic Award for Exemplary Online Learning Resource. Barker has been an invited presenter at 15 National Athletic Trainers' Association Annual Meeting and Clinical Symposium conferences.

Randy Deere, DA, AT-R

Dr. Randy Deere is a professor and program coordinator for the Graduate Sport Administration Program Athletic Administration Concentration at Western Kentucky University. Dr. Deere received his doctor of arts degree from Middle Tennessee State University in 1992, master of arts degree from Austin Peay State University in 1979, and a bachelor of science degree from Middle Tennessee State University in 1978. Dr. Deere spent 14 years as a collegiate athletic trainer before moving into university teaching. Dr. Deere's research interest focuses on online instructional pedagogy. Dr. Deere received the W. H. Mustaine Distinguished Service Award from the Kentucky Association of Health Physical Education Recreation and Dance (KAHPERD) in 2007, the University PE Teacher of the year award from KAHERD in 1998, and the WKU Faculty Service Award for the College of Health and Human Service in 2004. Dr. Deere has numerous national publications and presentations and served as *KAHPERD Journal* editor from 1993 until 2008. Additionally, Deere has served as a reviewer for Wolters Kluwer/ Lippincott Williams and Wilkins and created the PowerPoint supplements for *Applied Sports Medicine for Coaches* in 2009. He served as a Doping Control Officer for the United States Anti-Doping Agency from 2002 until 2008.

Part I

Basic Fundamentals

1 Taping Techniques, Wrapping Techniques for Support, and Protective Devices

Educational Objectives

Upon completing this chapter, the reader will be able to do the following:

- Explain philosophies and principles surrounding the proper use of adhesive and elastic tape and elastic wrap applications
- Select the proper supplies and specialty items used for taping, wrapping, or protective devices
- Describe the body preparation issues (for taping and wrapping) as they relate to hair removal, skin preparation, spray adherent, skin lubricants, and underwrap or cohesive tape
- Demonstrate correct application of taping wrapping and protective devices
- Explain the purposes for supportive wrapping techniques for anatomical joints and related structures

Introduction

The fundamentals of taping techniques, wrapping techniques for support, and protective devices are important to understand due to the increased population of active individuals. Scholars, health care professionals, and medical equipment specialists collaborated on this chapter to highlight the philosophies, identifications, applications, and other key components that revolve around taping techniques, wrapping techniques for support, and protective devices.

Proper Assessment of Injury

Before applying a preventive technique (tape, wrap, and/or device), a qualified physician or qualified health care professional should complete a proper injury evaluation. Following the injury evaluation, a qualified health care professional can then recommend proper taping techniques. This ensures that proper taping and wrapping techniques and protective devices are applied for support and stabilization. Also, developing a thorough knowledge of taping application fundamentals is imperative for the qualified health care professional.

Principles of Physical Rehabilitation

Supportive techniques, in conjunction with a rehabilitation program, enhance an individual's return to activity. Please note that taping and wrapping procedures are NOT a substitute for proper injury rehabilitation. You should follow specific instructions regarding injury rehabilitation and supportive taping and wrapping techniques and protective devices, as outlined by a qualified physician or qualified health care professional. You, as the qualified health care professional, need to develop a thorough knowledge of taping application fundamentals.

Fundamentals of Taping Procedures

1

Philosophies of Adhesive and Elastic Tape Application

With tape application, you must consider proper angle, direction, and tension. Adhesive tape is traditionally marketed as nonelastic, white tape. Currently, multiple colors exist in adhesive tape. Elastic tape has the ability to contract and expand and is commonly used in areas that need greater freedom of movement. Elastic tape also has the characteristics of conformability and strength. Additionally, it can be placed on the body part with fewer wrinkles and at unique angles. When you apply elastic tape, you must apply proper tension. The choice of adhesive or elastic tape in the application of a preventive technique is at your discretion.

Purpose of Taping

The primary purpose for tape application is to provide additional support, stability, and compression for the affected body part. Through proper application, taping techniques can be applied to shorten the muscle's angle of pull; to decrease joint range of motion; to secure pads, bandages, and protective devices; and to apply compression to control swelling. With the availability of commercial durable medical goods (braces and sleeves), you must have a comprehensive understanding of anatomy, physiology, and biomechanics, along with indications and contraindications of taping/wrapping versus bracing.

Medical Supplies: Adhesive, Elastic, and Cohesive Tape

The terms of choice for this text will be *adhesive tape*, *elastic tape*, and *cohesive tape*. Adhesive tape is traditionally marketed as nonelastic, white tape. Elastic tape provides greater freedom of mobility to the affected body part and is marketed as elastic tape. Both adhesive and elastic tapes are produced in a variety of widths. Cohesive (self-adherent) tape is a dressing material that will adhere to itself but not to other surfaces. This product comes in a variety of widths, lengths, and colors. Additionally, adhesive and elastic tapes are used to secure a wrap. In the preparation of some body parts, skin protection must be considered, such as a Band-Aid with a lubricant. The metric table is displayed for international conversion use.

METRIC TABLE

The metric table is displayed for international conversion use.

Inches	Centimeters	Inches	Centimeters
1	2.5	24	61
1.5	3.8	36	91.4
2	5.1	48	121.9
3	7.6	60	152.4
4	10.2	72	182.9
6	15.2	96	243.8
8	20.3	120	304.8
12	30.5		

inch x 2.54 = centimeter

centimeter x .39 = inch

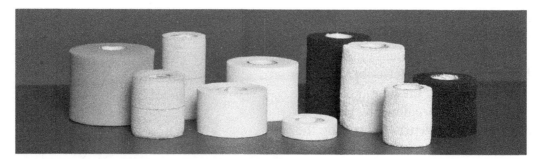

1

Selection of Proper Supplies and Specialty Items

One of the most critical aspects of taping techniques is the selection of proper supplies. Your selection depends on the number and types of sports or physical activities your organization offers and the frequency of injury in those activities. Purchasing supplies depends on budget, philosophy of medical staff regarding taping techniques, and occurrence of injury. Give special consideration to these additional supplies: benzoin (spray adherent), adhesive versus elastic tape, width of adhesive and elastic tape, cohesive tape, and length and width of elastic wraps.

Preparation of Body Part to Be Taped

In preparing the body for taping application, consider these six items:

1. **Removal of Hair (optional):** The individual should shave the affected body part. This will ensure a solid foundation for the tape, will allow for easy tape removal, and will reduce skin irritation.
2. **Clean the Area:** After hair removal, make sure the skin is clean and moisture free.
3. **Special Considerations:** Skin protection is important. Provide special care if the skin has allergies, tape or tape adherent, infections, or open and closed wounds.
4. **Spray Adherent (optional):** Spray the affected area with an adherent to aid in the adhesive quality.
5. **Skin Lubricants:** In areas of high friction or sensitivity, a skin lubricant such as a heel and lace pad will reduce the possibility of irritation.
6. **Underwrap or Cohesive Tape:** *Underwrap* is a foam wrap that is used when the individual is allergic to tape, whereas *cohesive tape* is a self-adherent tape that sticks to itself. Both of these products are used to hold heel and lace pads in place at high friction areas. The use of either underwrap or elastic tape over the entire taping area can compromise the stability of the taping technique. When applying an elastic wrap, do not use underwrap material.

Application and Removal of Taping Procedures

To tear tape, hold the adhesive or elastic tape firmly on each side of the proposed tear line. With proper tension applied on the tape, pull away the free end at an angle so that the force crosses the lines of the fabric and backcloth at a sharp angle. The tear then occurs sequentially through the backcloth. The more quickly you perform this maneuver, the more evenly tape edges will be torn. Some brands of elastic tape are extremely hard to tear by hand. Cut these elastic tape brands with scissors to ensure proper tape application and neatness.

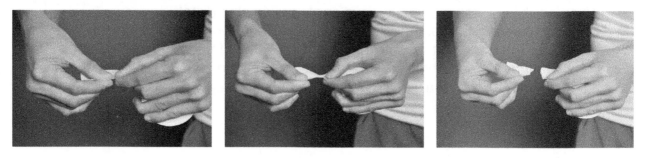

1

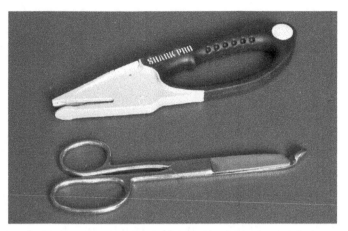

Remove adhesive and elastic tape easily by using bandage scissors or a specially constructed tape cutter. Apply a small amount of lubricant on the tip of the cutting device to allow the instrument to slip under the tape more readily, thus allowing you to remove the tape with ease. Avoid bony prominences by moving the scissor/cutter along the natural channels or in areas of greatest soft tissue cushion. Once you complete this, remove the tape from the skin in a constant and gradual manner. It is preferred that the tape be removed in the opposite direction from which it was applied. When pulling the tape from the skin at an angle of 180 degrees, exercise care to minimize removal of skin tissue and skin irritation. It is recommended that you apply pressure to the skin (pull the skin away from the tape), which will reduce the possibility of skin irritation. The daily use of a tape remover is recommended to help keep the skin clean and to prevent skin irritations and/or infections. Tape remover and/or alcohol will aid in the removal of tape mass and adherent from the skin.

TIPS FROM THE FIELD

Taping Procedures

- Know what body part and injury to which you are providing support and/or compression.
- Cover sensitive body parts (nail/nipple) and wounds with a protective covering.
- When applying a technique, learn to stand at a comfortable and stationary position and place the body part to be taped at your elbow height.
- When practicing, start with small length and width elastic wraps so you can learn common techniques such as figure of eight and joint spica. Once you have become proficient with wraps, then use adhesive and elastic tape.
- Apply proper tension to the tape so that circulation and neurological function will not be compromised.
- When applying a taping technique, follow the tape with your hand to smooth out all wrinkles.
- Overlap tape one half of its width to avoid spaces that could cause cuts and friction burns.
- Always angle the tape in order for the tape ends to meet at the anchor strips. If you do not succeed, retry the angle at a sharper degree.
- When applying closure strips, always apply proximal to distal.
- Upon completing the taping procedure, make sure you check for neatness and gaps, adequate support, and proper function of the affected area. In certain situations, the individual might be asked to perform function tests to establish appropriate technique application.
- **PRACTICE!**

Sport-Specific Rules on Taping

If you apply supportive techniques to an individual, you should be aware of specific rules governing tape application in that particular sport. Your application must fall within the guidelines established for each sport by appropriate governing bodies.

Precautions

Before you apply any techniques, the individual's skin temperature should be normal. To reduce the chance of skin irritation, after any therapeutic treatment, allow adequate time for the skin to return to its normal temperature. When applying support techniques, consider the safety of the individual your priority. Improper tape application can cause further injury. With all injured individuals, consult with a qualified physician. Do not use tape application with any disabling conditions.

Fundamental Procedures of Wrapping Techniques for Support

Philosophies of Elastic Wrap Application

Elastic wraps are primarily used to apply either compression or support to injured anatomical structures. Elastic wrap has the ability to contract and expand and is commonly used in areas that need greater freedom of movement. Elastic tape also has the characteristic of conformability and strength. As stated above, the selection of elastic wraps in the application of any preventive technique is at your discretion. You must develop a thorough knowledge regarding the fundamentals of the application of taping and wrapping procedures. During physical activity, supportive wraps are used to aid in muscle function and support and to reduce excessive range of motion. These applications are typically used in competition or practice. Spica wraps are traditionally employed at the hip and shoulder joints. Figure of eight wraps are placed over ankle, knee, elbow, and wrist and hand joints.

Purpose and Application of Elastic Wraps for Support

The primary purpose for the application of an elastic wrap is to provide support and/or compression for the affected body part. Through the proper application, wrapping techniques can be applied to shorten the muscle's angle of pull; to decrease joint range of motion; to secure pads, bandages, and protective devices; and to apply compression to reduce swelling. During physical activity, supportive wraps are used to aid in muscle function and support, reduce excessive range of motion, and aid in securing pads after the proper placement of felt, foam rubber, and protective devices. These applications are usually used for short periods, typically for competition or practice. Common terms for these wraps are *spica*, *figure of eight*, and *pad support*. Spica wraps are traditionally employed at the hip and shoulder joints. Figure of eight wraps are placed over ankle, knee, elbow, and wrist and hand joints.

Medical Supplies—Elastic Wrap

Elastic wrap is defined as a woven fabric that also allows for expansion and contraction and is used for compression or supportive techniques. This product is typically produced in 2-in., 3-in., 4-in., and 6-in. widths. In certain situations, an extra long length is more desirable. The ankle cloth wrap is a nonelastic cloth that is 2 in. wide and between 72 in. and 96 in. in length. Additionally, adhesive and elastic tape is used to stabilize the wrap. In the preparation of some body parts, consider skin protection, such as a Band-Aid with a lubricant. Depending on the number and types of sports or physical activities an organization offers and frequency of injury in those activities, a variety of supplies should be available. Purchasing

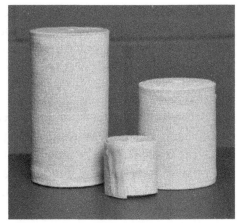

1

supplies depends on budget, philosophy of medical staff regarding taping techniques, and occurrence of injury. Also, give special consideration to benzoin (spray adherent) and the length and width of elastic wraps.

TIPS FROM THE FIELD

Wrapping Procedures

- Know what body part and injury to which you are providing support and/or compression.
- When applying a technique, learn to tape from a comfortable and stationary position and place the body part to be wrapped at your elbow height.
- When practicing, start with small length and width elastic wraps so you can learn common techniques such as figure of eight and joint spica.
- Apply proper tension to the wrap so that circulation and neurological function will not be compromised.
- When applying a wrapping technique, follow the wrap with your hand to smooth out all wrinkles.
- Overlap wrap one half of its width to avoid spaces that could cause cuts and friction burns.
- Upon completing the wrapping procedure, make sure you check for neatness and gaps, adequate support, and proper function of the affected area. In certain situations, the individual might be asked to perform function tests to establish appropriate technique application.
- When applying a compression wrap, always start distally and wrap proximally (toward the heart).
- **PRACTICE!**

Sport-Specific Rules on Wrapping

If you apply supportive techniques to an individual, you should be aware of specific rules governing supportive wrap application in that particular sport or physical activity. Your application must fall within the guidelines established for each sport by appropriate governing bodies.

Preparation of Body Part to Be Wrapped

In preparing the body for taping application, consider these three items:

1. **Clean the Area:** Make sure the skin is clean and moisture free.
2. **Special Considerations:** Skin protection is important. Provide special care if the skin has allergies, tape or tape adherent, infections, or open and closed wounds.
3. **Spray Adherent:** If needed, spray the affected area with an adherent to aid in the adhesive quality.

Proper Body Positioning

Before beginning a wrapping procedure, ask the individual to assume an anatomically correct and comfortable position. When applying a technique, stand at a comfortable and stationary position and place the body part to be taped and/or wrapped at your elbow height. The wrapping techniques presented in this text are the fundamental procedures. Variations can be achieved by adapting these techniques to a particular injury situation. Always give special consideration to the following:

- purpose of the wrapping procedure
- clinical application
- correct anatomical position
- appropriate supply selection

Note: A strong knowledge of anatomy, physiology, and biomechanics is essential.

Fundamentals of Protective Devices: Off-the-Shelf and Custom Braces

Philosophies of Protective Device

The use of a protective device can be highly beneficial to the particular body part if properly selected, applied, and worn. To avoid violating the manufacturer's specifications, follow the suggested guidelines for proper selection, application, and maintenance.

Definition of Protective Device

A protective device is a commercial product that is well designed and provides manufacturing liability and proper application instructions. The protective device is worn for protection, support, stability, or compression of an anatomical body part. Off-the-shelf braces are made in standard sizes and are available from merchandise in stock. In certain situations, these braces are called prefabricated braces. Custom braces are made to individual specification and fitted by qualified health care professionals and medical equipment specialists. Because these braces come in contact with the skin, it is highly recommended that daily maintenance should occur. As recommended by the manufacturer and Centers for Disease Control and Prevention (www.cdc.gov/mrsa/environment/athleticfacilities.html), proper steps in cleaning and disinfecting protective equipment should occur on a daily basis.

Purpose of Protective Device

The primary purpose for a protective device is to prevent an injury and to protect injured anatomical structures from further aggravation. Through proper application, a protective device can be applied to add additional protection, support, stability, and compression.

Protective Device: Sport-Specific Equipment, Liability, and Instruction

To ensure safety and product effectiveness, the protective device should have product liability coverage from the manufacturer and instructions for proper application. Sport-specific regulations, rules, and warnings exist concerning proper athletic equipment. Sport-specific equipment is worn as a standard uniform for participation in order to address individuals' safety. Standards of protection have improved through combined efforts of athletic governing bodies, the American Society for Testing and Materials (ASTM), the National Operating Committee on Standards for Athletic Equipment (NOCSAE), and the Hockey Equipment Certification Council (HECC).

Medical Device Authorization

As required, a qualified physician or qualified health care professional must prescribe a custom brace. Prior to this occurring, a qualified physician should complete a proper injury evaluation. Upon the physician's recommendation, a qualified health care professional and a medical equipment specialist can then recommend a custom or off-the-shelf protective device. This ensures that the proper device is applied for protection, support, stability, and/or compression. Also, the qualified health care professional and medical equipment specialist must develop a thorough knowledge of protective devices. See Figure 1.1 for an example of a Medco Sports Medicine Prescription Drug and Medical Device Authorization Form.

1

MEDCO
SPORTS MEDICINE
PRESCRIPTION DRUG & MEDICAL DEVICE
AUTHORIZATION FORM

If purchasing prescription pharmaceuticals, please complete sections A & B
If purchasing an Automated External Defibrillator (AED) unit or other medical device, please complete sections A & C

Dear Valued Customer,

In order to ship you prescription pharmaceuticals and/or medical devices, we must have authorization from a licensed physician or other authorized prescriber. This individual needs to fill out the form below and fax a copy of this page and a photocopy of their license to 800-222-1934.

If your School/Facility does not have a licensed physician or other authorized prescriber, but is licensed to purchase prescription pharmaceuticals and/or medical devices, please fax a copy of the license and this form for identification to 800-222-1934.

A) Name of School/Facility: _____

Attention:_____Customer #:_____

Address: _____

City & State:_____Zip:_____

Phone:_____Fax:_____

E-Mail:_____

B) I hereby authorize the internally designated representatives named below to order prescription products for this School/Facility. (please print)

1._____2._____

Type of authorization: ❏ Unlimited ❏ Limited (please attach list of products)

Physician/Authorized Prescriber Signature: _____

Physician/Authorized Prescriber Name (please print): _____

State License Number: _____
(please include photocopy of license)

C) I hereby acknowledge that I am aware that medical devices are intended for use by a physician or a person certified or trained to use such device.

Name (please print):_____

Title: _____

State License/Certification Number:_____

Signature:_____Date:_____

Rx Pharmaceuticals

Figure 1.1. Medco Prescription Drug and Medical Advice Authorization Form

Description of Protective Device

A variety of materials is used in the fabrication process of a protective device. The materials consist of different density and resilience. Low-density material absorbs force and high-density material disperses force. Resilience provides the ability to bounce or spring back into the position or shape after being stretched, impacted, or bent.

Selection of Proper Protective Device

The selection of a protective device is based on the optimal level of impacted intensity in regard to density, resilience, thickness, comfort, and specificity. In terms of appropriateness, consider age, size, skill level, and physical activity. Selecting a device that will absorb impact and disperse it before injury or stress occurs to the underlying body part is important. Because a variety of protective devices is available, a qualified physician or qualified health care professional and medical equipment specialist can determine whether the individual is best suited for an off-the-shelf or custom brace.

Application of Protective Device

The qualified health care professional, medical equipment specialist, and individual must be aware of the suggested guidelines, rules, and warnings when applying a protective device. Following the manufacturer's instructions is imperative, as is not modifying a device without a physician's approval. Once a device has been modified, the protection component is compromised, as the safety and liability to the manufacturer are no longer valid.

Precautions

Before applying any protective device, be aware of congenital deformities and scars that may alter the fit of the device. A protective device is an important product to prevent and protect injuries if used within the manufacturer's rules and guidelines. When you apply the support, safety should be your priority. Therefore, do not modify protective devices that are standardized and regulated. With all injured individuals, consult a qualified physician.

When a specialty pad is needed, consider the following criteria:

1. Does the pad meet specific rules and guidelines of the sport? If NO, then do not use the pad.
2. Does the pad perform the function for which it was designed? If NO, then do not use the pad.
3. Will the pad contribute to further injury to the area or to an adjacent area? If YES, then do not use the pad.
4. Will the pad alter the function or void the warranty of a manufactured piece of equipment (e.g., helmet, shoulder pads)? If YES, then do not use the pad.

Ask and answer these and other common questions routinely before having a specialty pad constructed.

Sport-Specific Rules on Braces and Special Devices

The use of braces and special devices is beneficial if they are intelligently selected, used in the appropriate setting, correctly fitted, properly applied, and used within the rules and guidelines of the specific sport. Qualified physician approval must be obtained prior to application and use. Three common specialty supplies used in braces and special devices techniques are listed below.

Foam. Whether adhesive or nonadhesive, foam can be used in conjunction with various taping/wrapping procedures to increase efficacy of the technique. Keep these items in mind prior to applying tape or wrap to foam: proper size, thickness, shape, and foam composition.

Felt. Apply this product with many of the same considerations as with foam rubber products. Factors that you should consider in the construction and application of a felt pad are size, varying thickness, and use of either adhesive or nonadhesive felt.

1

Thermoplastic. This rigid material could allow the injured individual to return to practice and/or competition with an increased awareness that the injury can be protected from further harm. Because of the hard composition of this product, thermoplastic material may be restricted from some sports, be limited to a certain body part, or require padding according to the guidelines of each sport.

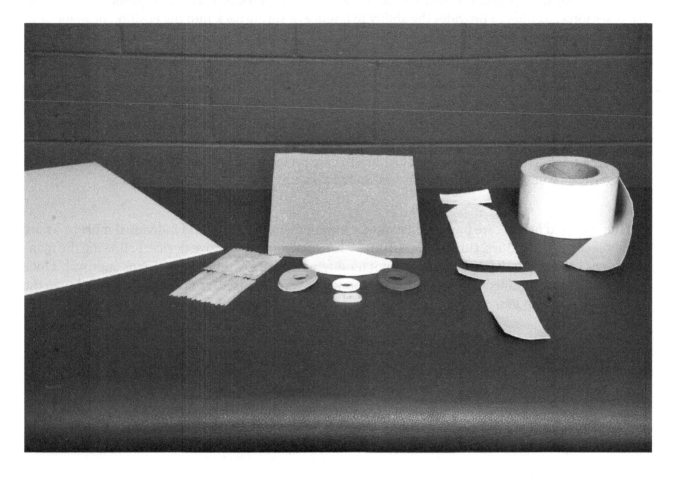

TIPS FROM THE FIELD

Protective Devices

- Educate individuals on the use, maintenance, applications, and limits of all protective devices worn.
- Use the manufacturer's sizing chart as a guide for proper application of a protective device.
- Daily inspect, dispose of, and/or repair protective devices.
- Monitor proper hygiene and maintenance to avoid abnormal infection or skin irritation.
- Inspect all protective devices before and after application to ensure safety.
- Do not distribute old, worn-out, ill-fitting protective devices to other players.
- Pad all protective materials sufficiently on the exterior to prevent injury to opposing individuals.

Anatomical Planes

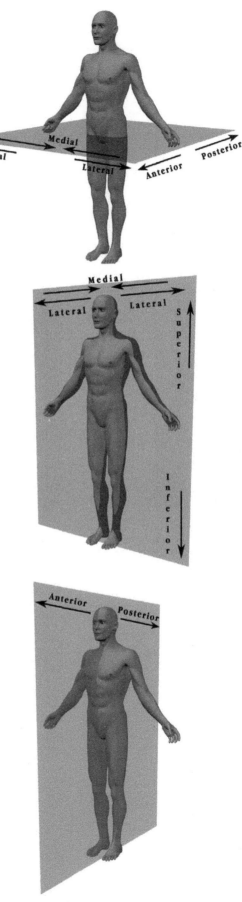

Transverse Plane. A horizontal plane at right angles to the vertical axis of the body. A plane that divides the body into a top and bottom portion.

Frontal Plane. A flat surface formed by making a cut, imaginary or real, through the body or a part of it. Planes are used as points of reference by which positions of parts of the body are indicated. In the human subject, all planes are based on the body being in an upright anatomical position.

Sagittal Plane. A vertical plane through the longitudinal axis of the body or part of the body, dividing it into right and left parts. If it is through the anteroposterior midaxis and divides the body into right and left halves, it is called a *median* or *mid-sagittal* plane.

2 Basic Fundamentals

Educational Objectives

Upon completing this chapter, the reader will be able to do the following:
- Explain philosophies and principles surrounding the proper use of elastic wrap applications for compression
- Demonstrate correct application of compression wraps and compression sleeves
- Explain the purpose and techniques for the application of compression wraps for the ankle, knee, elbow, wrist, and hand
- Explain philosophies and principles for casting and splinting

Introduction

The fundamentals of compression wrapping are necessary skills needed to properly administer injury care. An injury that occurs from a sprain, strain, or contusion will need immediate first aid attention to assist with the healing process. Compression to the injured area is a key part of the initial injury protocol and will help reduce swelling. A common acronym, PRICES (protection, rest, ice, compression, elevation, and support), lists the essential injury care measures. This chapter will discuss principles for injury care, fundamentals of compression wrapping, compression wraps, compression sleeves, casts, and splints.

Proper Assessment of Injury

Before applying a preventive technique (tape, wrap, and/or device), a qualified physician or qualified health care professional should complete an initial injury evaluation. Following initial injury evaluation, the professional can then recommend proper compression wrapping techniques. This ensures that proper wrapping techniques are applied for compression, support, and stabilization. Also, having a thorough knowledge of wrapping application fundamentals is imperative for the qualified health care professional. With specific written instruction (standing orders) provided by a qualified physician, the qualified health care provider's response to an acute injury should include the basic treatment protocol of protection, rest, ice, compression, elevation, and support (PRICES).

P (Protection). Once an injury has occurred, protect the injury from further damage by removing the individual from participation.

R (Rest). After the evaluation is completed, rest the injury. The length of rest is dependent on the severity of the injury; therefore, rest could easily be longer than 24 hours.

I (Ice). Apply cold to the injured area. This will aid in controlling bleeding and the associated swelling. The most common way to perform this activity is with an ice pack or plastic bags filled with ice covered with a towel. This treatment should be done for 10 minutes, with 3 hours in between treatment, four times per day. *Note:* Persons with known circulation problems must avoid ice. If problems arise, consult a qualified physician.

2

C (Compression). Using a compression wrap to control swelling, begin the elastic wrap distally (farthest from the heart) to the injury and spiral the wrap toward the heart on the involved extremity. Remove the wrap every 3 hours. *Note:* Compression wraps applied too tightly could interfere with circulation or nerve function. Signs and symptoms include extremities turning blue or pink, numbness and tingling of extremities, and increased pain. If the individual experiences this, remove the elastic wrap and reevalute the injury!

E (Elevation). Keep the injured body part elevated higher than the heart. This will allow gravity to keep excessive blood and associated swelling out of the injured area.

S (Support). Various techniques can be used to support an injury (i.e., elastic wrap, cohesive tape, first-aid equipment, or compression sleeve). If necessary, place the injured extremity in a first-aid splint. Examples of other supports include the use of crutches for a lower extremity injury or use of a sling for an upper extremity injury.

Fundamentals of Compression Wrapping Procedures

Philosophies of Elastic Wrap Application

Elastic wraps are primarily used to apply either compression or support to injured anatomical structures. The selection of elastic wrap, elastic tape, or cohesive tape for the application of compression to injured anatomical structure is at your discretion.

Medical Supplies: Compression Wrap, Cohesive Tape, and Compression Sleeve

Elastic wrap is defined as a woven fabric that allows for expansion and contraction and is used for compression and/or supportive techniques. Elastic wraps are manufactured in 2-in., 3-in., 4-in., and 6-in. widths and are usually 72 in. to 96 in. in length. In certain situations, an extra-long length is more desirable. Additionally, adhesive and elastic tapes are used to secure a wrap. Cohesive (self-adherent) tape is a dressing material that will adhere to itself but not to other surfaces. This product comes in a variety of widths, lengths, and colors. A compression sleeve is a commercial product that provides specific compression to anatomical structures (joints and muscles) and is usually sized from small to 4X-large.

METRIC TABLE

The metric table is displayed for international conversion use.

Inches	Centimeters	Inches	Centimeters
1	2.5	24	61
1.5	3.8	36	91.4
2	5.1	48	121.9
3	7.6	60	152.4
4	10.2	72	182.9
6	15.2	96	243.8
8	20.3	120	304.8
12	30.5		

inch x 2.54 = centimeter

centimeter x .39 = inch

Proper Body Positioning

Before beginning a wrapping procedure, ask the individual to assume an anatomically correct and comfortable position. When applying a technique, learn to stand at a comfortable and stationary position and place the body part to be wrapped at your elbow height. The wrapping techniques presented in this text are the fundamental procedures. Variations can be achieved by adapting these techniques to a particular injury situation. Always give special consideration to the

- purpose of the wrapping procedure
- clinical application
- correct anatomical position
- supply selection

Note: A strong knowledge of anatomy, physiology, and biomechanics is essential.

Precautions

Before applying a technique, make sure the individual's skin temperature is normal. To reduce the chance of skin irritation, after any therapeutic treatment, allow adequate time for the skin to return to its normal temperature. When applying support techniques, consider the safety of the individual your priority. With all injured individuals, consult a qualified physician.

TIPS FROM THE FIELD

Wrapping Procedures for Compression

- Know what body part and injury to which you are providing compression.
- When applying a compression wrap, always start distally and wrap proximally (toward the heart).
- When applying a technique, learn to stand at a comfortable and stationary position and place the body part to be wrapped at your elbow height.
- Apply proper tension to the tape so that circulation and neurological function will not be compromised.
- Follow the wrap with your hand to smooth out all wrinkles.
- Overlap the wrap one half of its width to avoid spaces that could cause cuts and friction burns.
- **PRACTICE!**

Compression Wraps: Elastic Wrap and Cohesive Tape

Developing a thorough knowledge regarding the fundamentals of the application of wrapping procedures is imperative. In applying a compression wrap, use a spiral pattern, and, beginning distal to the injury, wrap toward the heart. *On a frequent basis, remove the compression wrap to ensure that normal circulation and neurological function is present.

2

Ankle Compression–Elastic Wrap

Purpose: Compression

Supplies: 4-in. elastic wrap and 1½-in. adhesive tape

Wrapping Procedure:

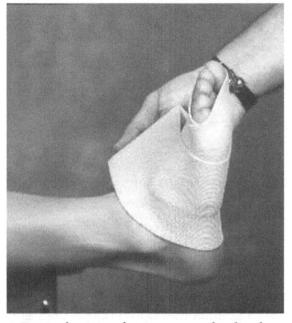

1. Begin the 4-in. elastic wrap at the distal part of the phalanges, spiral the wrap around the foot and ankle and on the distal aspect of the lower leg.

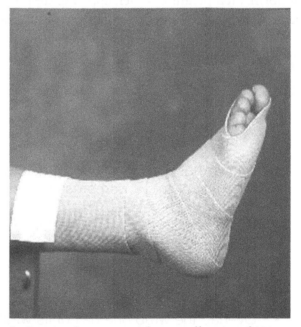

2. Secure the wrap with a small strip of 1½-in. adhesive tape.

Ankle Compression–Cohesive Tape

Purpose: Compression

Supplies: 2-in., 3-in., or 4-in cohesive tape and 1½-in. adhesive tape

Wrapping Procedure:

2

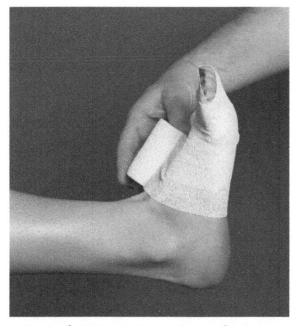

1. Begin the 2-in., 3-in., or 4-in. cohesive tape at the distal part of the phalanges, spiral the wrap around the foot and ankle and on the distal aspect of the lower leg.

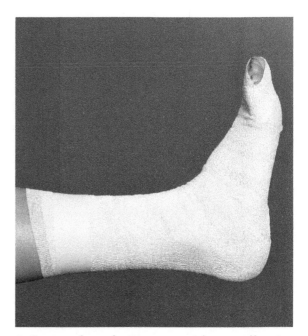

2. Secure the cohesive tape with a small strip of 1½-in. adhesive tape.

Knee Compression–Elastic Wrap

Purpose: Compression

Supplies: 6-in. extra long elastic wrap and 1½-in. adhesive tape

2

Wrapping Procedure:

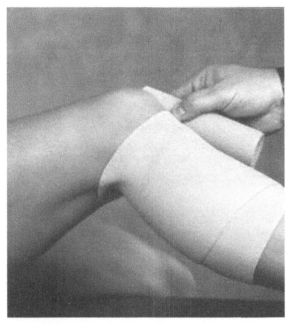

1. Begin the 6-in. elastic wrap around the lower leg, spiral around the leg, knee, and above the knee.

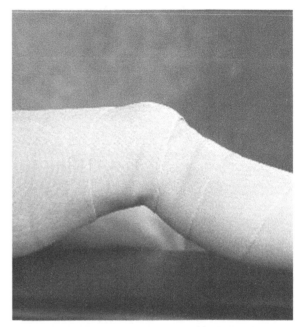

2. Secure the wrap with a small strip of 1½-in. adhesive tape.

Knee Compression–Cohesive Tape

Purpose: Compression

Supplies: 3-in, 4-in., or 6-in. cohesive tape and 1½-in. adhesive tape

Wrapping Procedure:

2

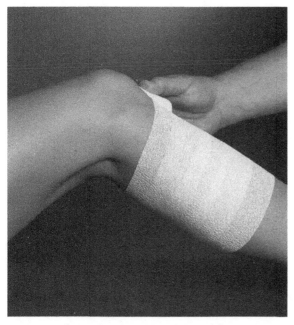

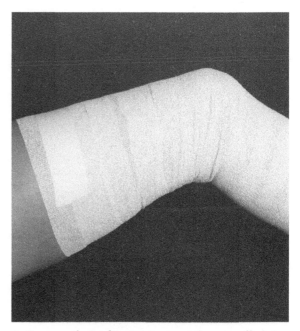

1. Begin the 3-in, 4-in., or 6-in. cohesive tape around the lower leg, spiral around the leg, knee, and above the knee.

2. Secure the cohesive tape with a small strip of 1½-in. adhesive tape.

Elbow Compression–Elastic Wrap

Purpose: Compression

Supplies: 6-in. elastic wrap and 1½-in. adhesive tape

2

Wrapping Procedure:

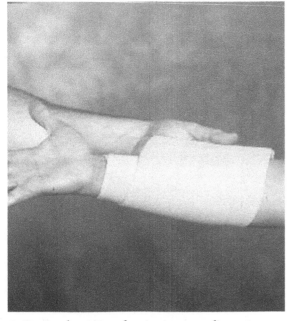

1. Begin the 6-in. elastic wrap at the wrist, spiral the wrap around the forearm and above the elbow joint.

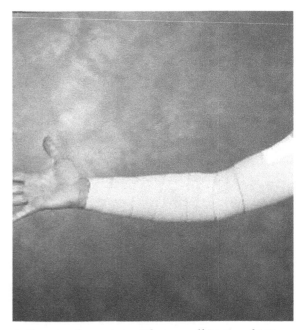

2. Secure the wrap with a small strip of 1½-in. adhesive tape.

Elbow Compression–Cohesive Tape

Purpose: Compression

Supplies: 3-in. or 4-in. cohesive tape and 1½-in. adhesive tape

Wrapping Procedure:

2

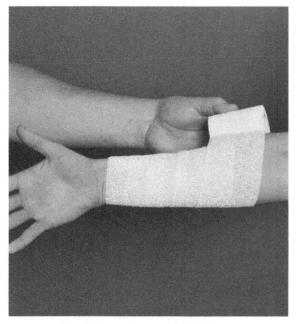

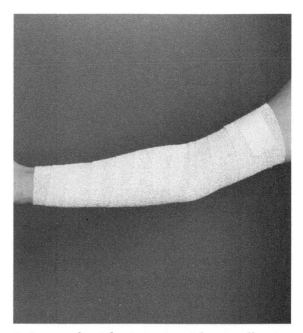

1. Begin the 3-in. or 4-in. cohesive tape at the wrist, spiral the wrap around the forearm and above the elbow joint.

2. Secure the cohesive tape with a small strip of 1½-in. adhesive tape.

Wrist/Hand Compression Elastic Wrap

Purpose: Compression

Supplies: 4-in. elastic wrap and 1½-in. adhesive tape

2

Wrapping Procedure:

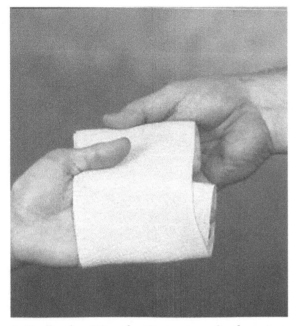

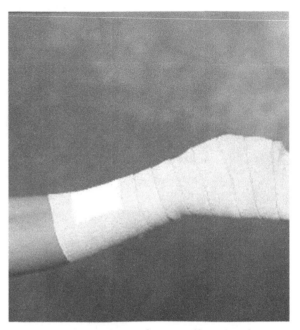

1. Begin the 4-in. elastic wrap at the finger tips, spiral around the hand and above the wrist.

2. Secure the wrap with a small strip of 1½-in. adhesive tape.

Wrist/Hand Compression–Cohesive Tape

Purpose: Compression

Supplies: 2-in. or 3-in. cohesive tape and 1½-in. adhesive tape

Wrapping Procedure:

2

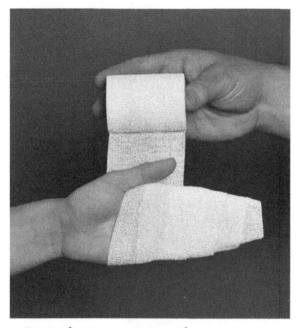

1. Begin the 2-in. or 3-in. cohesive tape at the finger tips, spiral around the hand and above the wrist.

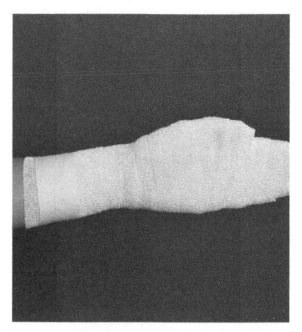

2. Secure the cohesive tape with a small strip of 1½-in. adhesive tape.

Compression Sleeves

Compression sleeves are garments designed to provide pressure to upper and lower body extremities. They may be used for prevention, support, swelling reduction, and to increase circulation. The Stromgren Nano Flex Supports were manufactured for comfortable support and compression. They are odor free, antibacterial, and wicks moisture away from the body. The negative ions enhance the body's natural healing process for individuals. In addition, the infrared rays help increase blood circulation and the retention of body heat.

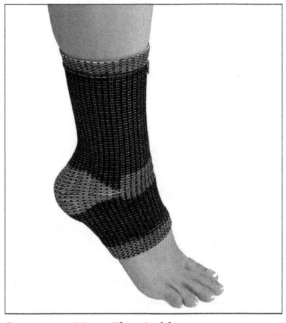

Stromgren Nano Flex Ankle

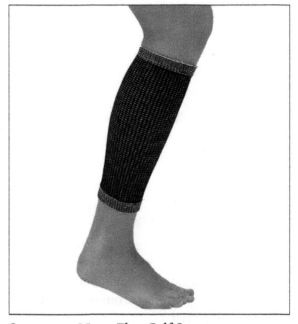

Stromgren Nano Flex Calf Support

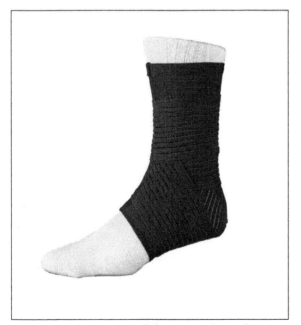

Stromgren Model 329 Heel-Lock
Ankle Support

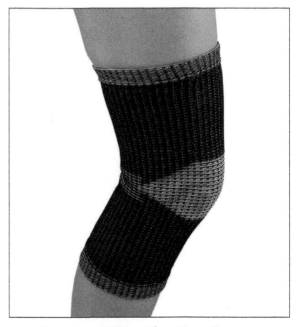

Stromgren Nano Flex Knee Support

2

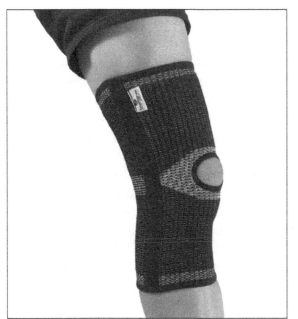

Stromgren Nano Flex Open Patella Knee Support With Spiral Stays

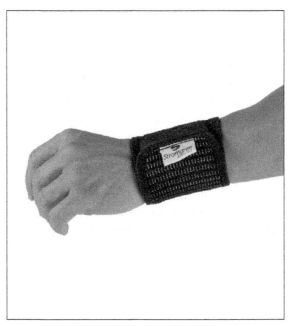

Stromgren Nano Flex Wrist

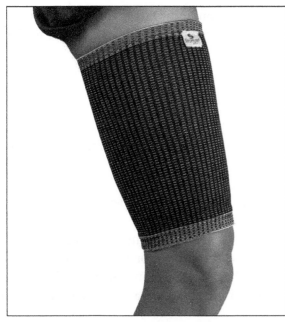

Stromgren Nano Flex Thigh Support

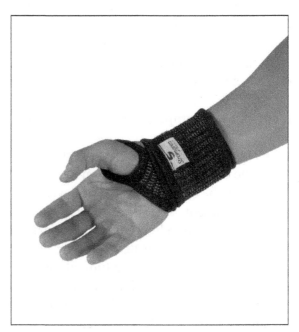

Stromgren Nano Flex Wrist and Thumb

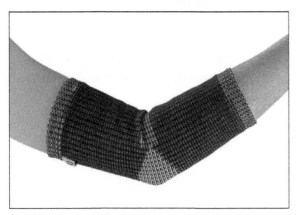

Stromgren Nano Flex Elbow Support

Casts and Splints

2

An individual who has sustained an injury and requires a cast or splint should be aware of possible complications associated with the use of these immobilization techniques. The most pressing issue is the possibility of developing compartment syndrome. Compartment syndrome is a true orthopedic medical emergency in which delayed treatment could result in permanent functional loss or loss of limb. Compartment syndrome is caused by an increase in pressure within fascial compartments of the forearm and lower leg. This increase in pressure is due to swelling as a result of the body's natural response to injury, lack of elevation of the injured extremity, splint and cast applications that are applied too tightly, or a combination of these factors. Elevated intracompartmental pressure leads to a reduction in venous outflow, which increases interstitial pressure and results in tissue necrosis. Six hours after the development of compartment syndrome, complete functional recovery cannot be guaranteed, and beyond 8 to 12 hours, the damage is irreversible. Qualified health care professionals, coaches, individuals (patient), and parents (if applicable) should be educated about the symptoms of compartment syndrome:

- Pain: A steady increase of pain out of proportion to the injury. Pain sensation is greater than that experienced at the time of injury.
- Pressure: Cast or splint has the sensation of "being too tight."
- Paresthesia: An abnormal or unpleasant sensation that results from injury to one or more nerves. It is often described by patients as numbness and tingling or as a prickly, stinging, or burning feeling; sensation of tingling, burning, or prickling.
- Pulselessness: Weak or absence of distal pulse.

If any of these symptoms are present, take the following steps:

1. Contact the provider and advise them of the symptoms. If the provider cannot be reached, proceed to the closest emergency room for evaluation.
2. Elevate the extremity above the level of the heart.
3. If the patient is wearing a splint, loosen the compressive dressing that is securing the splint. Loosening can relieve pressure while maintaining immobilization.
4. If the patient is wearing a cast, bi-valve the cast to relieve pressure. Bi-valving is making complete (proximal to distal) longitudinal cuts on the cast to relieve pressure. (For the Qualified Health Care Professional: A short arm cast should be cut on both the dorsal area and the ventral area and the short leg cast should be cut on both the medial area and the lateral area. Be sure to use a cast spreader to "pop" the cast open.)

Generally, these steps may relieve acute symptoms of compartment syndrome; however, the provider must evaluate the individual even if the symptoms subside.

Splint: Splints should be used in the acute setting (injury greater than 7 to 10 days postinjury) as opposed to casts because splints can accommodate for swelling commonly associated with injuries. Be sure to evaluate neurovascular status before and after splint application.

Materials:
- cast padding (cotton or synthetic)
- compressive wrap
- bandage tape to secure the compressive wrap

- water to activate the splint resin
- bandage scissors
- splint material: fiberglass cast tape or plaster cast material (prefab = Ortho-glass)

Be sure to use the appropriate size when selecting these materials. The width of the individual's hand is a good indicator of which size should be used. The use of stockinette is contraindicated due to its compressive effect, which may add to the potential of compartment syndrome.

Cast: Individuals should be transitioned into a cast after the acute phase (injury greater than 7 to 10 days postinjury) for proper immobilization. Be sure to evaluate neurovascular status before and after cast application.

Materials:
- stockinette
- cast padding (cotton or synthetic)
- fiberglass or plaster cast tape
- water to activate the cast resin
- bandage scissors

Be sure to use the appropriate size when selecting these materials. The width of the individual's hand is a good indicator of which size should be used.

Part II

Techniques for Lower Extremities

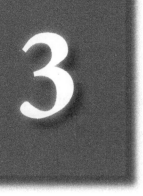

Foot, Ankle, and Lower Leg

Educational Objectives

Upon completing this chapter, the reader will be able to do the following:
- Identify anatomical landmarks critical for correct taping procedures
- Describe the purpose for the applications of adhesive and elastic tape
- Select the proper supplies and specialty items used for taping
- Explain the steps in preparing the body for taping, wrapping or protective device
- Describe and demonstrate the purposes, clinical applications, anatomical structures, supplies needed, pre-taping and taping procedures for anatomical areas
- Identify the proper use and application of protective devices for the foot, ankle, and leg

Introduction

Lower extremity injuries related to the foot, ankle, and lower leg represent a large population. Knowing the basic concepts will prove beneficial for proper injury management. This chapter will improve insight by addressing the terminology, taping techniques, wrapping techniques, protective devices, and musculoskeletal disorders related to the ankle, foot, and lower leg.

Terminology

Dorsal. Upper surface (e.g., top of foot).

Plantar. Ventral aspect of the foot (sole of the foot).

Proximal. Closest to the midline or center of the trunk; nearest to the point of attachment, origin, or other point of reference.

Distal. Away from a center, from the midline, or from the trunk. A point that is greater from point of reference (opposite of proximal).

Plantar flexion. Act of drawing the toe or foot toward the plantar aspect of the proximally conjoined body segment; opposite of dorsiflexion.

Dorsiflexion. Act of drawing the toe or foot toward the dorsal aspect of the proximally conjoined body segment.

Inversion. Act of rotating the pronated foot internally on the ankle; turning the sole of the foot inward.

Eversion. Act of rotating the pronated foot externally on the ankle; turning the sole of the foot outward.

Pronation. Act of rotating the hand or foot internally on its long axis; medial rotation of the forearm, as in turning the palm of the hand downward.

Supination. Act of rotating a hand or foot externally on its long axis; lateral rotation of the forearm, as in turning the palm of the hand upward.

Malleolus. A rounded bony protuberance on each side of the ankle joint.

Pes cavus. High arch; deformities of the foot.

Pes planus. Flat feet.

Stirrup. Any U-shaped loop or piece.

Heel lock. Commonly used in ankle taping, this supportive technique aids in stabilizing the calcaneus; medial and lateral heel locks are usually applied.

Figure of eight. Bandaging of a joint where the initial turn circles the one part of the joint and the second turn circles the adjoining part of the joint to form a figure of eight.

Foot, Ankle, and Lower Leg

Taping Techniques and Protective Devices

Developing a thorough knowledge regarding the fundamentals of the application of taping/wrapping procedures is imperative. Review Chapter 1 before applying any technique.

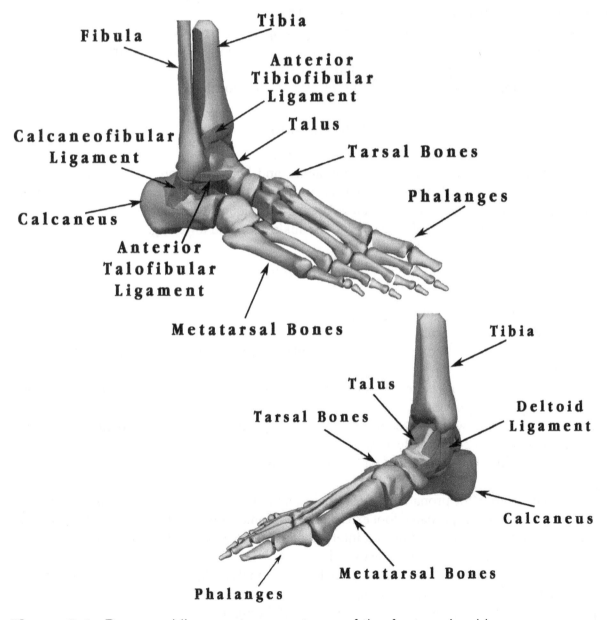

Figure 3.1. Bony and ligamentous anatomy of the foot and ankle

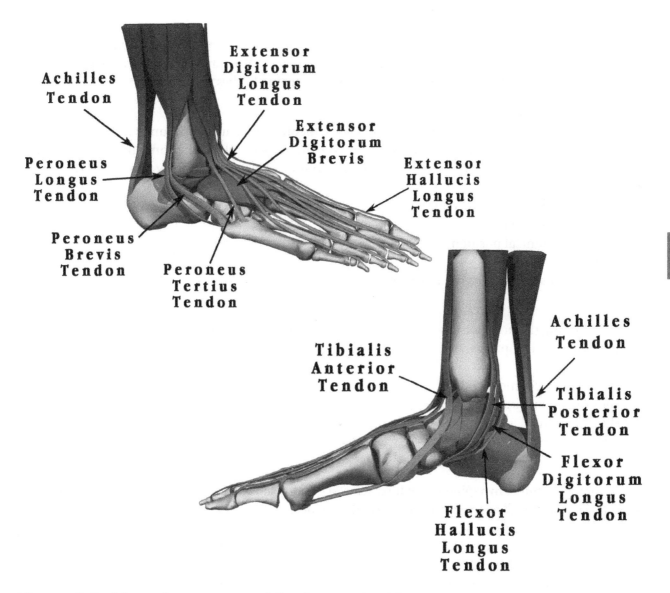

Figure 3.2. Muscular anatomy of the foot and ankle

Proper Assessment of Injury

Before applying a preventive technique (tape, wrap, and/or device), a qualified physician or qualified health care professional should complete a proper injury evaluation. Following injury evaluation, the professional can then recommend proper taping techniques. This ensures that proper taping techniques are applied for support and stabilization. Also, developing a thorough knowledge of taping application fundamentals is imperative for the professional.

Purpose and Application of Adhesive and Elastic Tape

The primary purpose for tape application is to provide additional support and stability for the affected body part. Through proper application, taping techniques can be applied to shorten the muscle's angle of pull; to decrease joint range of motion; to secure pads, bandages, and protective devices; and to apply compression to reduce swelling.

Medical Supplies and Specialty Items

Purchasing supplies depends on budget, philosophy of medical staff regarding taping techniques, and occurrence of injury. Review Chapter 1 before applying any technique.

Specific Rules on Taping, Wrapping, and/or Protective Device

If you apply supportive techniques to an individual, you should be aware of specific rules governing tape application in that particular sport or physical activity. Your application must fall within the guidelines established for each sport by appropriate governing bodies.

Special Techniques: Adjunct Taping Procedures

The taping techniques presented are the fundamental procedures. Adjunct techniques will be shown to provide additional support; however, you should still follow the fundamental procedures. Variations can be achieved by adapting these techniques to a particular injury situation. Always give special consideration to

- purpose of the taping procedure
- clinical application
- correct anatomical position
- supply selection
- tape/wrap technique or protective device

Preparation of Body Part for Taping

In preparing the body for tape application, consider these six items:
1. removal of hair (optional)
2. clean the area
3. special considerations
4. spray adherent (optional)
5. skin lubricants
6. underwrap or cohesive tape

Proper Body Positioning

Before beginning any taping procedure, select a comfortable table height and ask the individual to assume an anatomically correct and comfortable position.

- Neutral Position of Foot: When taping the foot, the anatomical position should be slightly plantar flexed (10 to 15 degrees).
- Neutral Position of Ankle Joint: With the leg fully extended, the foot should be positioned at a 90-degree angle.

When applying a technique, learn to stand at a comfortable and stationary position and place the body part to be taped at your elbow height.

Taping Techniques

The taping techniques presented are the fundamental procedures. A strong knowledge of anatomy, physiology, and biomechanics is essential. Developing a thorough knowledge regarding the fundamentals about the application of taping/wrapping procedures is imperative. Review Section A - Chapter 1 before applying any technique.

When applying tape to the foot or ankle, pull the tape lateral to avoid excessive tension/compression on the fifth metatarsal.

Great Toe–Dorsal

Purpose:	To limit excessive motion of the first metatarsophalangeal joint (MP Joint), therefore helping to prevent or stabilize a sprain or turf toe
Clinical Application:	Sprain to first metatarsophalangeal joint (turf toe)
Anatomical Structure:	First metatarsal joint (great toe)
Anatomical Position:	Ankle should be placed in neutral position and first MP joint placed in neutral position
Supplies:	1-in. or 1½-in. adhesive tape, and 2-in. elastic tape

3

Taping Procedure:

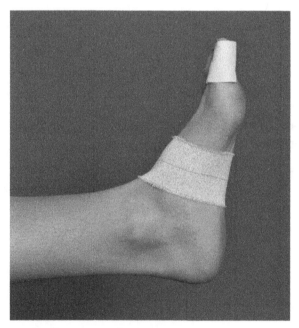 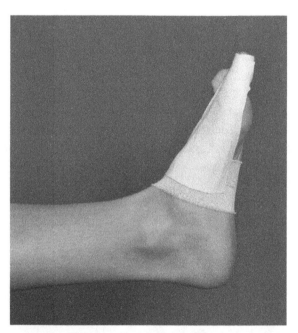

1. Apply two anchor strips.
a. Apply adhesive anchor strip around distal aspect of the great toe.
b. Apply elastic anchor strip around the mid-foot. This strip should begin on the dorsal aspect, go lateral, and continue across the plantar aspect to the mid-foot medial portion, crossing the tape ends.

2. Apply four to six strips of adhesive tape to form a fan shape. This will provide adequate support. Place fan-shaped tape from the anchor on the great toe, covering the affected dorsal area and ending on the elastic anchor at the mid-foot.

3

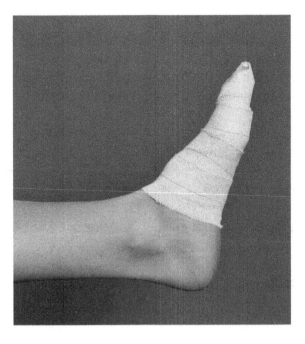

3. Using a continuous strip of elastic tape, apply a figure of eight around the great toe and mid-foot. This will aid in abduction of the first MP joint and should assist in preventing excessive movement, flexion, or extension of the MP joint.

*Upon completion of the procedure, make sure you check for neatness and gaps, adequate support, along with proper function of the affected area. In certain situations, the individual might be asked to perform function tests to establish appropriate technique.

These adjunct taping procedures can be used in conjunction with the basic technique presented.

Adjunct Technique A. Apply two circular strips of adhesive tape, around the proximal and distal aspect of first and second phalanges. This is commonly referred to as buddy taping.

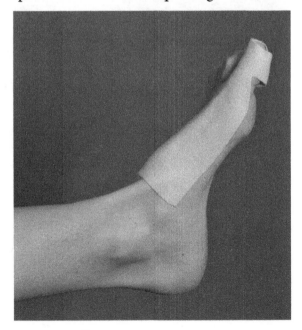

Adjunct Technique B. Apply a strip of moleskin over the Dorsal area.

Great Toe–Plantar

Purpose:	To limit excessive motion of the first metatarsophalangeal joint (MP Joint), therefore helping to prevent or stabilize a sprain or turf toe
Clinical Application:	Sprain to first metatarsophalangeal joint (turf toe)
Anatomical Structure:	First metatarsal joint (great toe)
Anatomical Position:	Ankle should be placed in neutral position and first MP joint placed in neutral position
Supplies:	1-in. or 1½-in. adhesive tape, and 2-in. elastic tape

3

Taping Procedure:

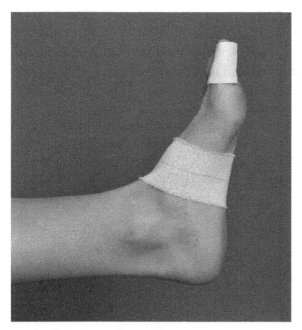

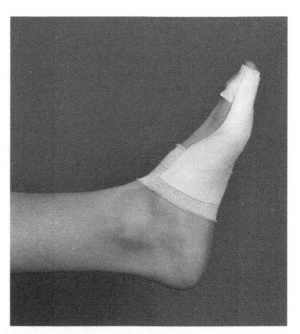

1. Apply two anchor strips.
a. Apply adhesive anchor strip around distal aspect of the great toe.
b. Apply elastic anchor strip around the mid-foot. This strip should begin on the dorsal aspect, go lateral, and continue across the plantar aspect to the mid-foot medial portion, crossing the tape ends.

2. Four to six strips of adhesive tape should be applied to form a fan shape. This will provide adequate support. Place fan-shaped tape from the plantar aspect of the anchor on the great toe, covering the affected plantar area and ending on the elastic anchor at the mid-foot.

3

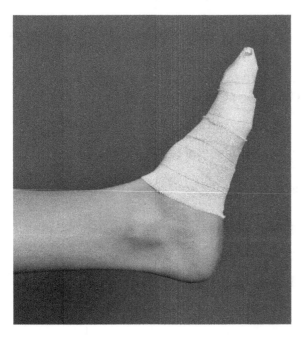

3. Using a continuous strip of elastic tape, apply a figure of eight around the great toe and mid-foot. This will aid in abduction of the first MP joint and should assist in preventing excessive movement, flexion or extension of the MP joint.

*Upon completion of the procedure, make sure you check for neatness and gaps, adequate support, along with proper function of the affected area. In certain situations, the individual might be asked to perform function tests to establish appropriate technique.

These adjunct taping procedures can be used in conjunction with the basic technique presented.
Adjunct Technique A. Apply two circular strips of adhesive tape, around the proximal and distal aspect of first and second phalanges. This is commonly referred to as buddy taping.

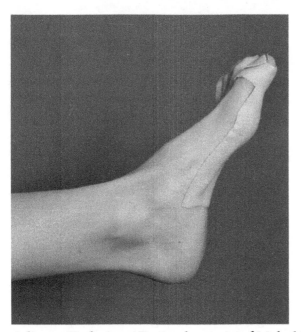

Adjunct Technique B. Apply a strip of Moleskin over the plantar area.

Heel

Purpose:	To provide compression and support to the calcaneus fat pad and underlying tissue
Clinical Application:	Contusion to the heel area
Anatomical Structure:	Calcaneus (Heel)
Anatomical Position:	Place ankle joint in neutral position
Supplies:	1-in. or 1½-in. adhesive tape
Pre-Taping Procedures	Apply tape adherent to affected area

3

Taping Procedure:

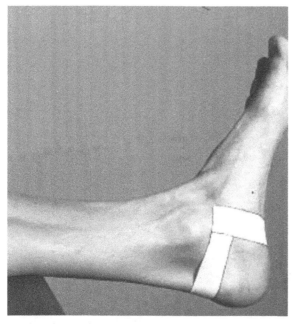

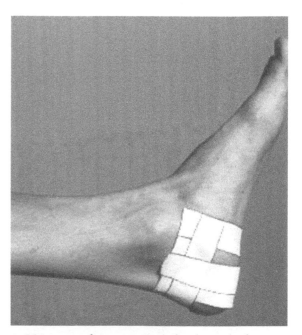

1. Apply anchor strips (medial to lateral) to enclose affected heel area.
a. Across the heel (plantar surface).
b. Around the heel (posterior surface).

2. Using an alternative method, apply four to six strips of tape that apply direct pressure to the heel. Overlap these support strips one half of the tape width. The tape should be applied proximal to distal on the plantar surface of the foot.

3

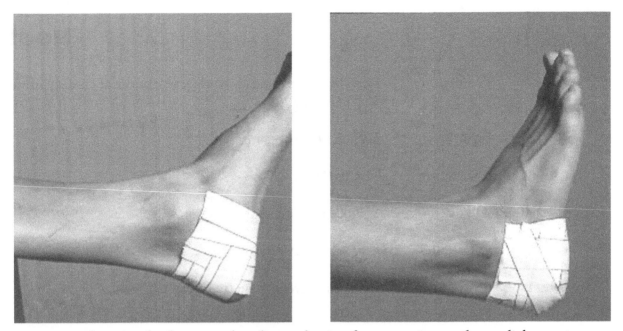

3. To cover the entire heel area, apply a diagonal strip of tape starting on the medial aspect, crossing the heel, and ending on the lateral aspect.

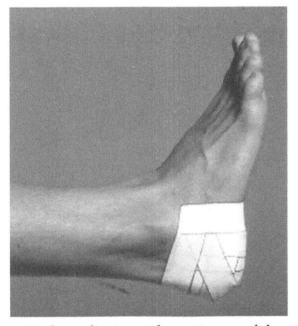

4. To close, place an anchor strip around the heel, from the medial to lateral side of the foot.

*Upon completion of the procedure, make sure you check for neatness and gaps, adequate support, along with proper function of the affected area. In certain situations, the individual might be asked to perform function tests to establish appropriate technique.

Metatarsal Arch

Purpose:	To elevate the metatarsal heads
Clinical Application:	Dropped metatarsals, contusions, strains, and sprains
Anatomical Structure:	Metatarsal arch
Anatomical Position:	Ankle should be positioned in a slight plantar flexed position
Supplies:	¼-in. or ½-in. felt, 2-in. or 3-in. elastic tape, and 1½-in. adhesive tape

3

Pre-Taping Procedure:

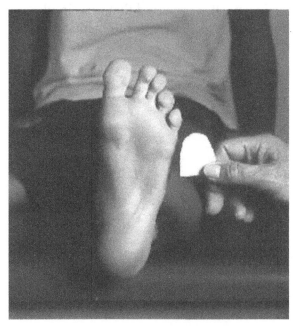

First, cut a ¼-in. or ½-in felt piece in a diamond shape (metatarsal pad) with all sides slightly tapered.

Taping Procedure:

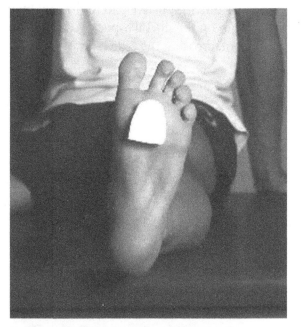

1. Place the metatarsal pad proximal to the heads of the second through fourth metatarsals.

3

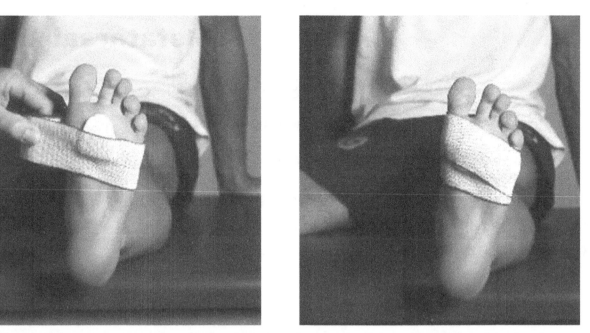

2. Secure this supportive pad to the foot by using elastic tape. It is preferred that this circular strip begin on the dorsal aspect, go lateral, and continue across plantar aspect to medial portion of the foot, crossing the tape ends.

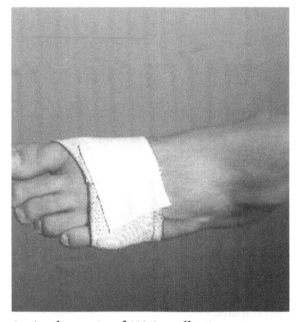

3. Apply a strip of 1½-in. adhesive tape over the tape ends to secure the elastic tape.

*Upon completion of the procedure, make sure you check for neatness and gaps, adequate support, along with proper function of the affected area. In certain situations, the individual might be asked to perform function tests to establish appropriate technique.

Medial Longitudinal Arch

Purpose:	To support the bones, ligaments, muscles, and accessory components on the plantar surface of the foot
Clinical Application:	Arch sprains, shin splints, and common overuse injuries
Anatomical Structure:	Plantar surface of the foot
Anatomical Position:	Ankle should be positioned in a slight plantar flexed position.
Supplies:	1-in. and 1½-in. adhesive tape, 2-in. elastic tape, and heel and lace pad
Pre-Taping Procedures:	Place the heel and lace pad over the individual's posterior aspect of the heel

3

Taping Procedure:

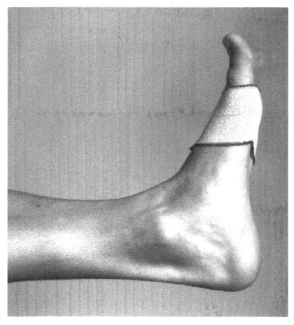

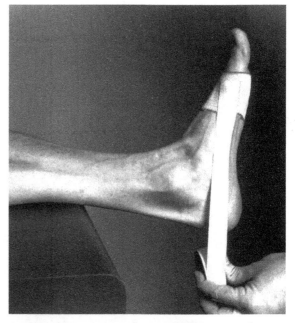

1. Place an anchor strip of 2-in. elastic tape around the metatarsals. This circular strip should begin on the dorsal aspect, go lateral, and continue across the plantar aspect to the medial portion of the foot, crossing the tape ends.

2. Next, starting at the medial aspect of the first MP joint, apply 1-in. adhesive tape along the medial margin of the foot and around the heel, pulling diagonally across the plantar surface and ending on the medial aspect of the first MP joint.

3

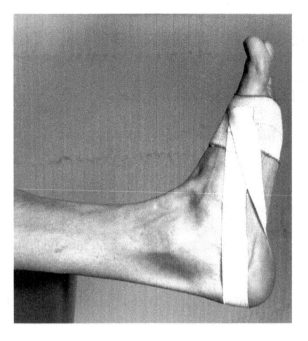

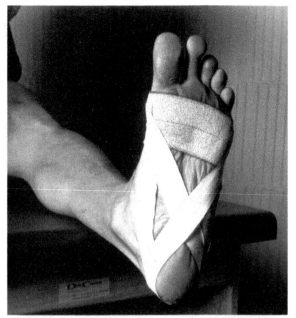

3. Start at the lateral aspect of the fifth MP joint and place a strip of 1-in. adhesive tape on the outside of the foot and around the heel, pulling diagonally across the plantar surface and going back to the lateral aspect of the fifth MP joint. Repeat steps 2 and 3. Remember to overlap the tape one half of its width.

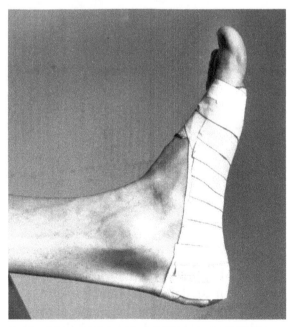

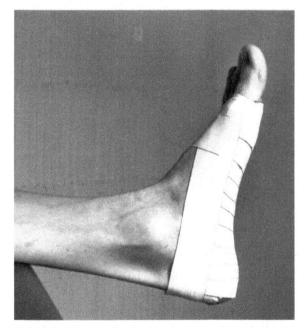

4. Starting at the proximal aspect of the foot, apply strips of tape from the lateral to medial side. The tape strips should cover the entire plantar surface of the foot. This should provide additional support to the inner longitudinal arch.

5. To close, apply a 1½-in. adhesive anchor strip from the medial aspect of the first metatarsal, around the heel, and to the lateral aspect of the fifth metatarsal head.

*Upon completion of the procedure, make sure you check for neatness and gaps, adequate support, along with proper function of the affected area. In certain situations, the individual might be asked to perform function tests to establish appropriate technique.

Adjunct Taping Procedure: Medial Longitudinal Arch

This adjunct taping procedure can be used in conjunction with the basic technique presented.

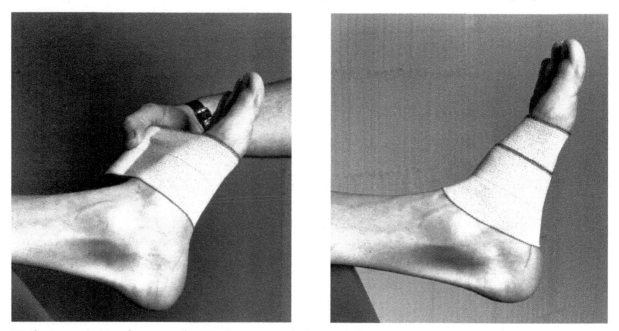

Technique A: Apply 3-in. elastic tape around the mid-foot area. It is preferred that this circular strip begin on the dorsal aspect, go lateral, and continue across the plantar aspect to the medial portion of the foot, crossing the tape ends.

3

Toe Splint

VIDEO

Purpose:	To aid and support the injured phalanx
Clinical Application:	Contusions, sprains, and strains to the phalanges of the foot
Anatomical Structure:	Phalanges
Anatomical Position:	Neutral position
Supplies:	½-in. adhesive tape and gauze, felt, and/or foam rubber
Pre-Taping Procedures:	Cut gauze, felt, or foam rubber to appropriate size

3

Taping Procedure:

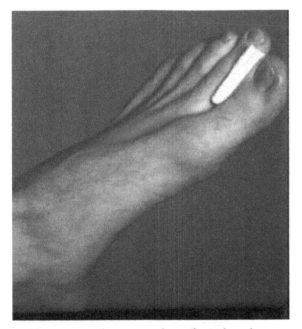

1. Place gauze between the affected and adjacent phalanges.

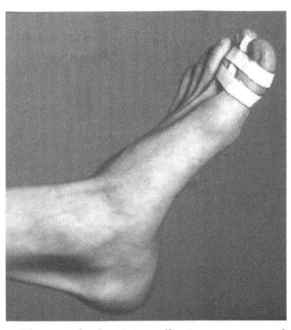

2. Then apply the ½-in. adhesive tape around both phalanges. This technique is known as buddy taping.

*Upon completion of the procedure, make sure you check for neatness and gaps, adequate support, along with proper function of the affected area. In certain situations, the individual might be asked to perform function tests to establish appropriate technique.

Plantar Fasciitis

Purpose:	To aid in the reduction of stress on the plantar fascia and related foot structures
Clinical Application:	Plantar fasciitis
Anatomical Structure:	Plantar surface of the foot
Anatomical Position:	Ankle placed in a slightly plantar flexed position
Supplies:	3-in. adhesive felt (moleskin), 2-in. elastic tape, and 1½-in. adhesive tape

3

Pre-Taping Procedure:

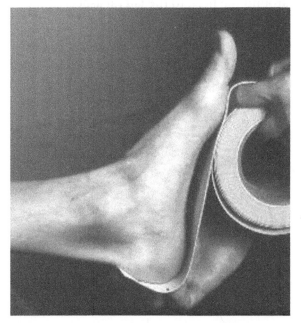

Before you begin, cut the adhesive felt to the length that measures from the metatarsal heads to the posterior aspect of the heel.

Taping Procedure:

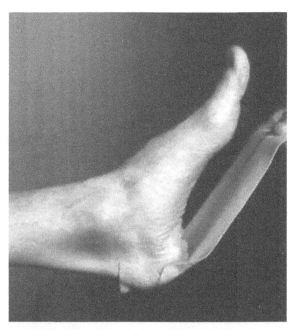

1. With the ankle slightly plantar flexed, apply the adhesive felt strip at the posterior aspect of the heel and firmly pull toward the metatarsal heads. To eliminate binding, cut a V on both edges of the adhesive felt where the felt crosses the heel area. Once adequate tension is applied, press the adhesive felt against the plantar aspect of the foot.

3

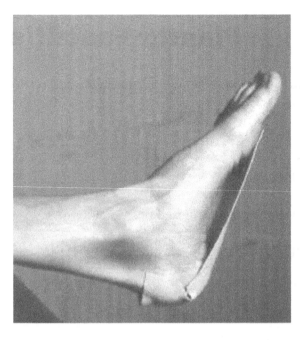

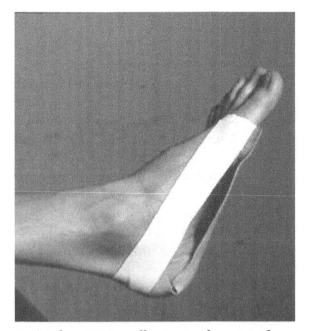

2. Apply a 1½-in. adhesive anchor strip from the medial aspect of the first metatarsal, around the heel, to the lateral aspect of the fifth metatarsal head.

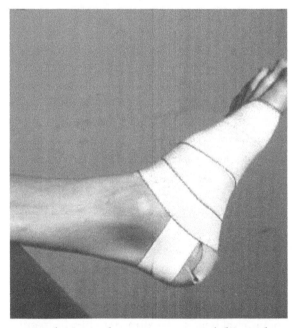

3. Apply 2-in. elastic tape around the mid-foot area. This circular strip should begin on the dorsal aspect, go lateral, and continue across the plantar aspect to the medial portion of the foot, crossing the tape ends.

*Upon completion of the procedure, make sure you check for neatness and gaps, adequate support, along with proper function of the affected area. In certain situations, the individual might be asked to perform function tests to establish appropriate technique.

Adjunct Taping Procedures: Plantar Fasciitis
These adjunct taping procedures can be used in conjunction with the basic technique presented.

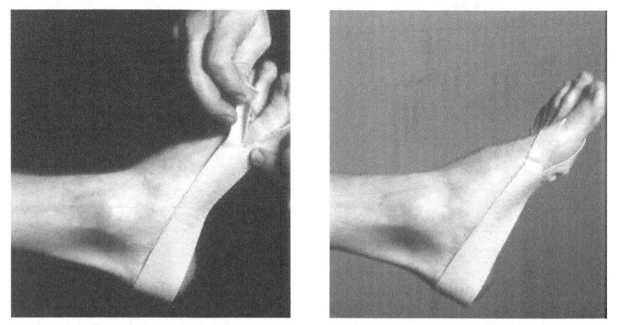

Technique A. The individual should be instructed to slightly plantar flex the ankle and flex the phalanges. Apply a 2-in. adhesive felt anchor strip from the medial aspect of the first metatarsal head, around the heel, to the lateral aspect of the fifth metatarsal head (allow 1 in. additional length on both ends of this strip). Split both ends of this strip of moleskin lengthwise approximately 2 in., and place the ends of the tape on the dorsal and plantar aspect of the first and fifth metatarsals.

3

3

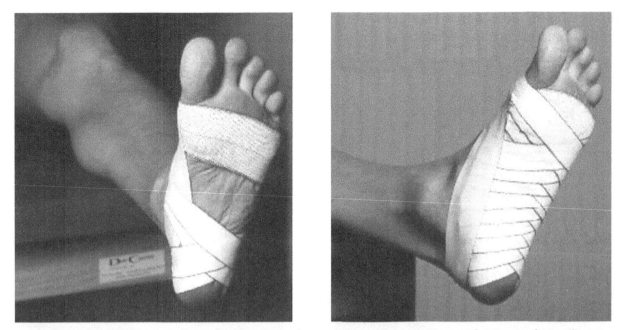

Technique B: The X-pattern technique. Apply a 1½-in. adhesive tape anchor strip from the medial aspect of the first metatarsal head, around the heel, to the lateral aspect of the fifth metatarsal head. Place an anchor strip of 2-in. elastic tape around the head of the metatarsals (lateral to medial). It is preferred that this circular strip begin on the dorsal aspect, go lateral, and continue across the plantar aspect to medial portion of the foot, crossing the tape ends. Starting at the proximal aspect of the foot (heel), apply strips of 1-in. adhesive tape in a diagonal fashion (45 degrees). Alternate the application of the 1-in. strips from lateral to medial, and vice versa. Cover the entire plantar surface of the foot with the tape strips. Apply a closure strip of 1½-in. adhesive tape from the medial aspect of the first metatarsal head, around the heel, to the lateral aspect of the fifth metatarsal head.

Ankle–Closed Basket Weave

Purpose:	To support and stabilize the ankle joint for INVERSION sprains
Clinical Application:	Sprains
Anatomical Structure:	Ankle joint
Anatomical Position:	Ankle joint in neutral position
Supplies:	1½-in. or 2-in. adhesive tape and heel and lace pads

3

Pre-Taping Procedure:

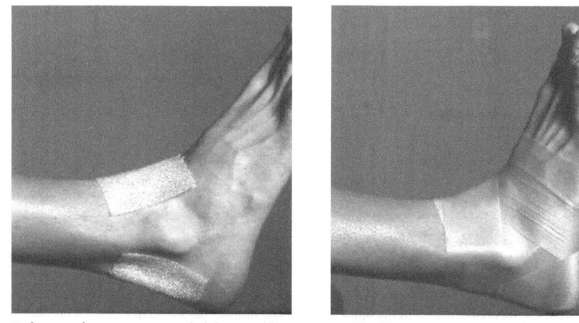

Before you begin taping, apply lubricated heel and lace pads at high friction areas: one at the distal aspect of the Achilles tendon and the other at the dorsal aspect of the ankle joint. Additionally, apply underwrap to secure the two heel and lace pads in place and reduce skin irritation. It is critical that the foot remain at a 90-degree angle for this procedure.

Taping Procedure:

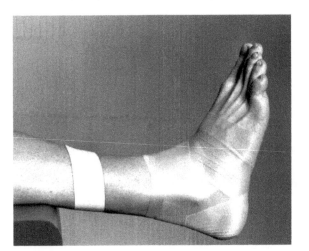

1. Apply an adhesive tape anchor strip around the lower leg at approximately the musculo-tendon junction of the gastrocnemius. Because the leg at this site is not cylindrically shaped, angle the tape slightly to conform to the leg.

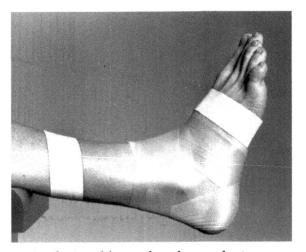

2. Apply an additional anchor at the instep. Remember that excessive tension on the fifth metatarsal could cause pain on weight bearing.

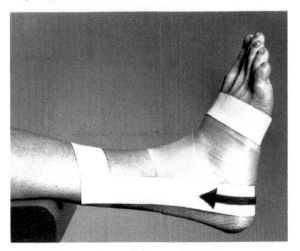

3. Apply the first of three stirrup strips. Beginning on the medial aspect of the upper anchor, continue this stirrup down the inside of the leg, over the medial malleolus, across the plantar aspect of the foot, over the lateral malleolus, and up the lateral aspect of the leg, ending at the lateral aspect of the upper anchor. Apply proper tension to cause some eversion of the foot, thus helping to reduce inversion.

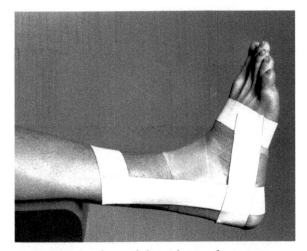

4. Apply the first of three horseshoe strips. The first horizontal strip is started on the medial aspect of the foot, continues toward the heel and below the medial malleolus, crosses the Achilles tendon below the lateral malleolus, and ends on the lateral aspect of the foot.

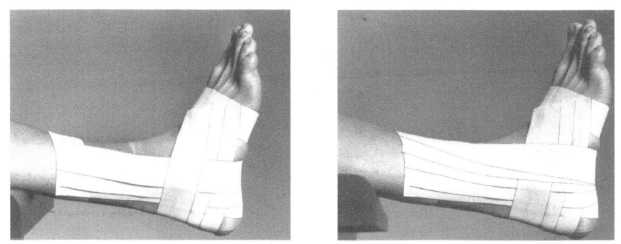

5. Repeat Steps 3 and 4 twice, overlapping the tape one half of its width. These interlocking strips should provide additional support for this technique. The completed portion of this closed basket weave has sets of interlocking stirrups and horseshoe strips. Apply a proximal anchor for support. For proper adherence, apply compression to the tape so that the tape conforms to the body part.

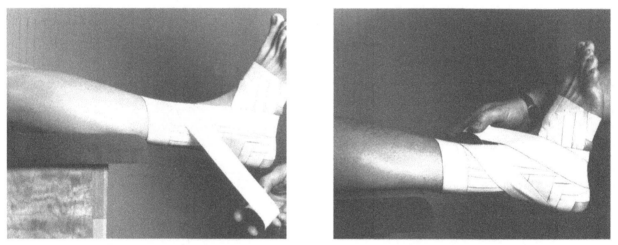

6. Apply the first heel lock strip. Begin on the anterior portion of the upper anchor, continuing down the outside of the leg, crossing the Achilles tendon around the medial aspect of the heel, angling underneath the foot, and moving up the lateral aspect of the leg. Apply proper tension to ensure stabilization of the calcaneus.

3

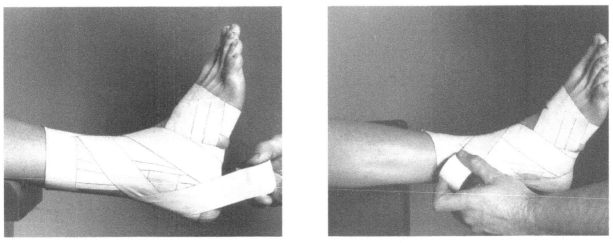

7. Apply the second heel lock strip. Begin on the anterior portion of the upper anchor, continuing down the inside of the leg, crossing the Achilles tendon around the lateral aspect of the heel, angling underneath the foot, and moving up the medial aspect of the leg.

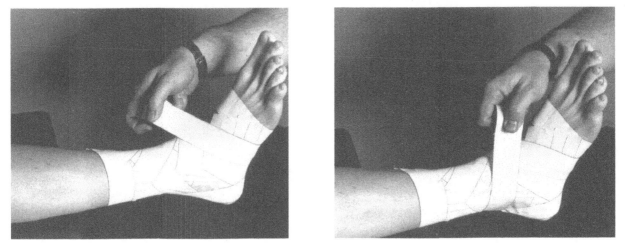

8. Apply a figure of 8. Starting on the dorsal aspect of the foot, move medially down the inside of the foot, across the plantar portion, up the outside of the foot to the starting point. Continue medially around the lower leg, crossing the Achilles tendon and finishing at the origin of this figure of 8 technique. By encircling the foot and leg, this technique will assist in dorsal flexion and eversion.

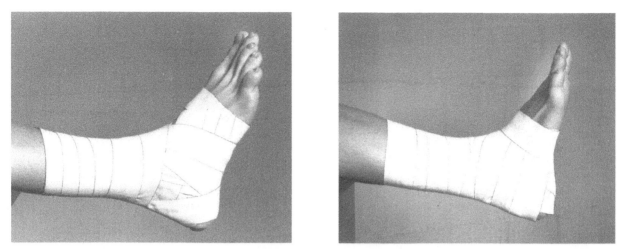

3

9. Apply final closure strips. Begin proximally and work distally. From the upper anchor, apply individual circular strips around the extremity to cover tape ends. Make sure you overlap the tape approximately one half of its width on each strip.

*Upon completion of the procedure, make sure you check for neatness and gaps, adequate support, along with proper function of the affected area. In certain situations, the individual might be asked to perform function tests to establish appropriate technique application.

Adjunct Taping Procedures: Ankle

These adjunct taping procedures can be used in conjunction with the basic technique presented.
Technique A. In conjunction with the stirrups, you can apply adhesive felt prior to the adhesive tape for additional support. Apply this from the medial to the lateral aspect.

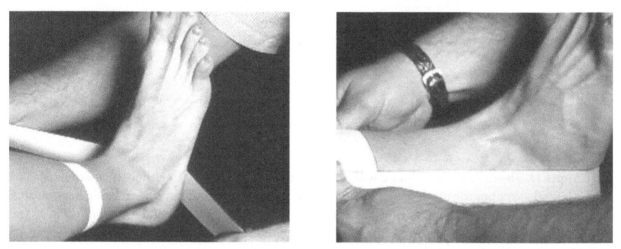

Technique B. In certain situations, joint trauma could be present on both the medial and lateral aspects of the ankle joint. It is recommended that the stirrups be placed on the plantar portion of the heel with equal tension applied both medially and laterally and/or tension bilaterally prior to attachment on the upper anchor.

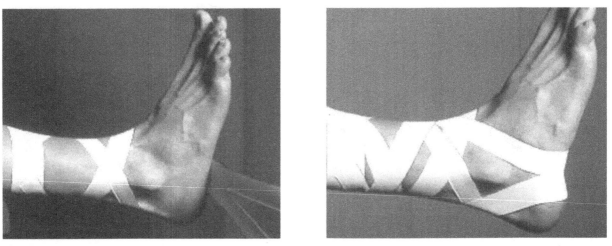

3

Technique C. This technique is known as the Spartan technique. Using 2-in. adhesive tape, approximately 24 in. to 30 in. in length, place the middle portion of this stirrup strip on the plantar portion of the heel. Split each end approximately 10 in. to 12 in. Starting on the medial side, place the first half strip below and in front of the medial malleolus and spiral up the leg. Place the second half of that strip below and behind the medial malleolus and spiral up the leg. Repeat this procedure on the lateral side. Two to three strips of adhesive tape with the Spartan technique can provide additional stability to ankle joint.

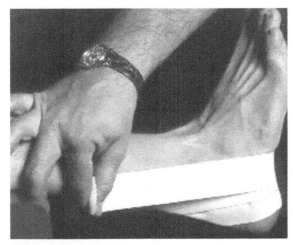
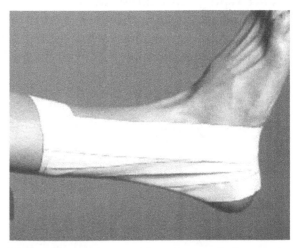

Technique D. The Side Bar technique will provide additional support to either the medial aspect or the lateral aspect of the ankle joint. Using 1½-in. adhesive tape, anchor lateral side bars on the medial aspect of the foot, angling underneath the foot, moving up the lateral aspect of the leg, and ending on the upper anchor. Depending on the size of the foot and severity of the injury, apply four to eight overlapping side bar strips.

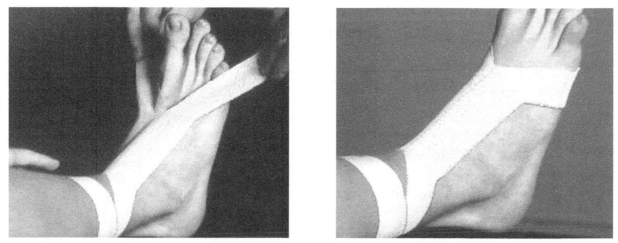

3

Technique E. The dorsal check rein aids in preventing the ankle joint from excessive plantar flexion. Using 3-in. elastic tape, cut a strip 12 in. to 15 in. in length, split both ends lengthwise approximately 4 in. With the ankle in neutral position, encircle the leg with one of the split ends, pulling the tape to full tension. Encircle the mid-foot region with the other split ends of the elastic tape.

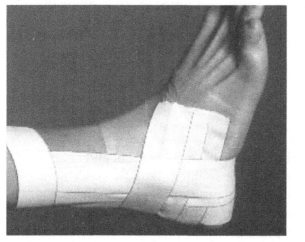
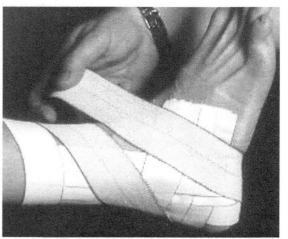

Technique F. In the combined elastic and adhesive tape technique, using 2-in. elastic tape, apply heel locks and figure of 8 in a continuous fashion.

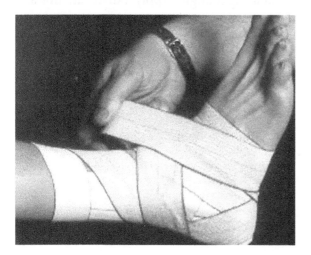

Ankle–Open Basket Weave

3

Purpose:	To provide compression and support to the ankle joint while allowing room for expansion due to swelling. This technique is commonly used for acute ankle injury treatment.
Clinical Application:	Acute ankle sprain
Anatomical Structure:	Ankle joint
Anatomical Position:	Ankle joint in neutral position
Supplies:	1½-in. or 2-in. adhesive tape and 4-in. elastic wrap
Pre-Taping Procedures	After hair removal, make sure the skin is clean and moisture free. Skin protection is important. Provide special care if the skin has allergies, infections, or open and closed wounds. Spray the affected area with an adherent to aid in the adhesive quality and provide stability to the supportive technique.

Taping Procedure:

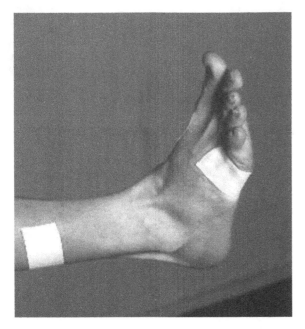

1. In this application, leave a 1-in. gap on the anterior aspect of the foot and ankle to allow for swelling. With the ankle joint in a neutral position, apply an adhesive tape anchor strip around the lower leg at approximately the musculo-tendon junction of the gastrocnemius. Because the leg at this site is not cylindrically shaped, apply the tape at a slight angle. Apply a distal anchor at the instep.

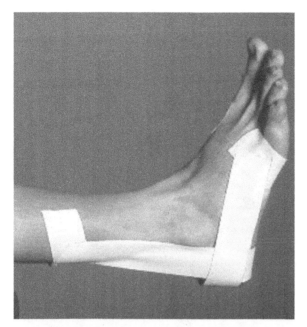

2. Apply the first stirrup strips. Beginning on the medial aspect of the upper anchor, continue this stirrup down the inside of the leg, over the medial malleolus, across the plantar aspect of the foot, and up the lateral aspect of the leg, ending at the lateral aspect of the upper anchor. Apply proper tension to prevent ankle inversion.

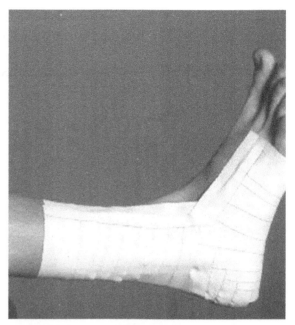

3. Apply the first horseshoe strips. The first horizontal strip is started on the medial aspect of the foot, continues toward the heel and below the medial malleolus, and crosses the Achilles tendon, ending on the lateral aspect of the foot. Remember to overlap the tape one half of its width, repeat steps 2 and 3. These interlocking strips provide additional support. Also, cohesive tape can be used to provide compression

3

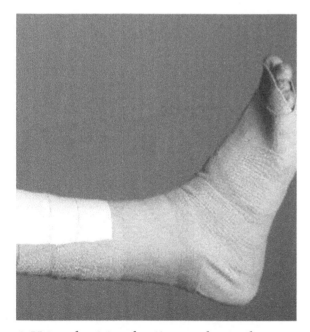

4 Using the 4-in. elastic wrap, begin the wrap at the distal part of the phalanges, spiral the wrap around the foot and ankle and up the leg. Secure the wrap with a small strip of adhesive tape. Also, cohesive tape can be used to provide compression.

*Upon completion of the procedure, make sure you check for neatness and gaps, adequate support, along with proper function of the affected area. In certain situations, the individual might be asked to perform function tests to establish appropriate technique.

3

Adjunct Taping Procedure: Open Basket Weave
These adjunct taping procedures can be used in conjunction with the basic technique presented.

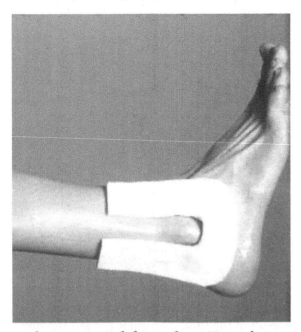

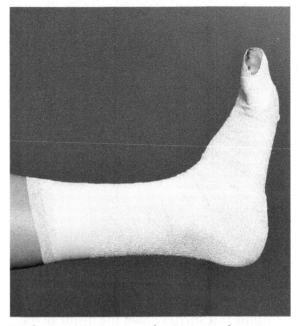

Technique A: Felt horseshoe. To apply additional compression to the lateral aspect of the ankle joint, construct a horseshoe out of ½-in. felt. Placement of this horseshoe is around the lateral malleolus, with the open ends of the horseshoe pointing upward and the curve of the horseshoe just distal to the malleolus. Then apply the open basket weave taping technique over the felt horseshoe.

Technique B. Using cohesive tape, begin the wrap at the distal part of the phalanges, spiral the wrap around the foot and ankle and up the leg.

Shin Splint

Purpose:	To help reduce the pain associated with shin splints
Clinical Application:	Shin splints (medial tibial stress syndrome)
Anatomical Structure:	Lower leg, ankle, and foot
Anatomical Position:	Knee should be fully extended and ankle joint slightly plantar flexed.
Supplies:	½-in. or ⅜-in. felt and 1½-in. adhesive tape
Pre-Taping Procedures:	Cut felt in 1-in. x 6-in. strip

3

Taping Procedure:

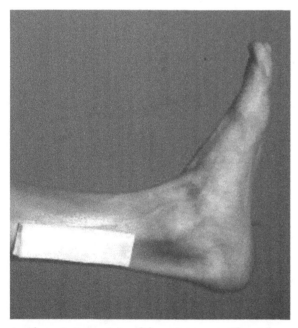

1. Place 1-in. x 6-in. felt strip over affected area.

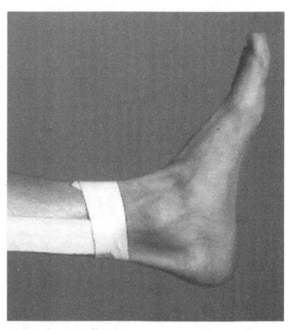

2. Apply an adhesive tape strip. Begin the tape 1 in. to 2 in. below the distal end of the felt pad, proceed laterally, cross the Achilles tendon, and pull the tape and felt back against the tibia. Tear the tape.

3

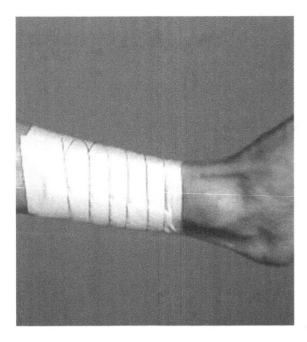

3. Apply four to six additional overlapping adhesive tape strips as applied in step 2. *Special Consideration:* This taping technique is for pain on the medial aspect of the tibia. For pain on the lateral side of the tibia, pull the tape in the opposite direction.

*Upon completion of the procedure, make sure you check for neatness and gaps, adequate support, along with proper function of the affected area. In certain situations, the individual might be asked to perform function tests to establish appropriate technique.

Adjunct Taping Procedures: Shin Splint
These adjunct taping procedures can be used in conjunction with the basic technique presented.

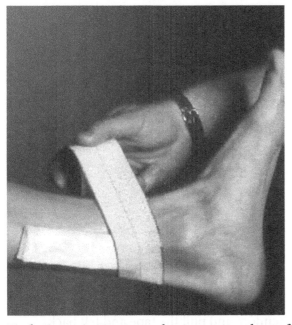

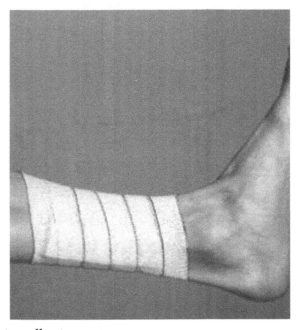

Technique A. Use 2-in. elastic tape in place of 1½-in. adhesive tape.

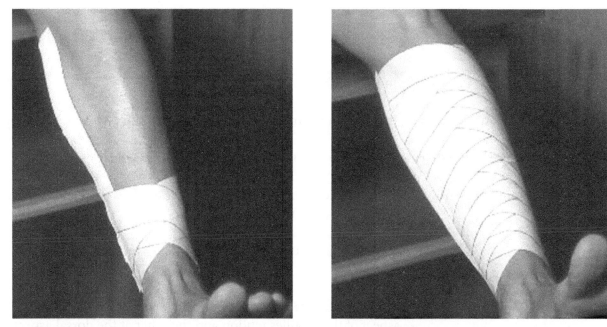

3

Technique B: The X-pattern technique. Apply two vertical anchor strips, approximately 6 in. to 10 in. in length, over the medial and lateral aspects of the leg. Begin at the medial anchor, cross the anterior aspect at a 45-degree angle, and end on the lateral anchor. Apply the second strip from the lateral anchor, crossing the anterior aspect at a 45-degree angle and ending on the medial anchor. Repeat this step seven to nine times, overlapping the tape by one half of its width. Place a final anchor over each original anchor to help hold the tape in place. Do not cover the posterior aspect of the leg with adhesive tape.

Achilles Tendon

Purpose:	To reduce the stress on the Achilles tendon
Clinical Application:	Tendinitis and strains of Achilles tendon and posterior lower leg
Anatomical Structure:	Achilles tendon, gastrocnemius, and soleus muscles
Anatomical Position:	With individual in prone position, the ankle is placed in plantar flexion and knee in slight flexion.
Supplies:	1½-in. adhesive tape, 3-in. elastic tape, ½-in. felt, and heel and lace pads
Pre-Taping Procedures:	Apply heel and lace pads at high friction areas: one at the distal aspect of the Achilles tendon and the other at the dorsal aspect of the ankle joint.

Taping Procedure:

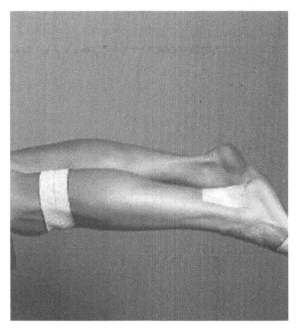

1. Apply two anchors using 3-in. elastic tape. Apply the proximal anchor on the proximal aspect of the gastrocnemius. Apply the distal anchor around the heads of the metatarsals (ball of the foot). It is preferred that this circular strip begin on the dorsal aspect, go laterally, and continue across the plantar aspect to medial side of the foot, crossing the tape ends.

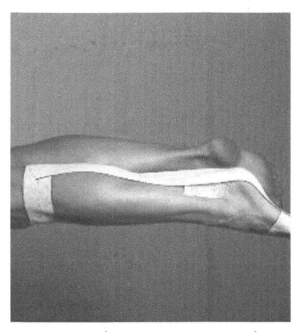

2. Using 3-in. elastic tape, measure on the posterior aspect the distance between the proximal and distal anchors. This will be the length required for your support strips. Apply the first support strip of elastic tape, going from the proximal anchor to the distal anchor. Upon application, apply full tension to the tape ends. Note that slight knee flexion and plantar flexion is maintained so that there is a small degree of tension across this first support strip.

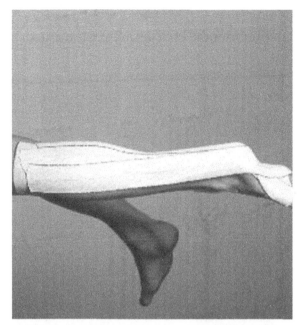

3. Apply additional strips of support in an angular fashion to cover the posterior aspect of the leg and the plantar aspect of the foot. For proper adherence, apply compression to the tape so that the tape conforms to the body parts.

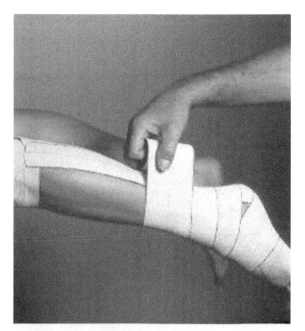

4. Using 3-in. elastic tape, close up the procedure by overlapping the tape by one half of its width on each revolution.

3

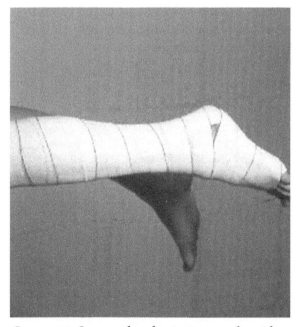

Comment: Secure the elastic tape ends with anchors of 1½-in. adhesive tape.

*Upon completion of the procedure, make sure you check for neatness and gaps, adequate support, along with proper function of the affected area. In certain situations, the individual might be asked to perform function tests to establish appropriate technique.

3

Adjunct Taping Procedure: Achilles Tendon
This adjunct taping procedure can be used in conjunction with the basic technique presented.

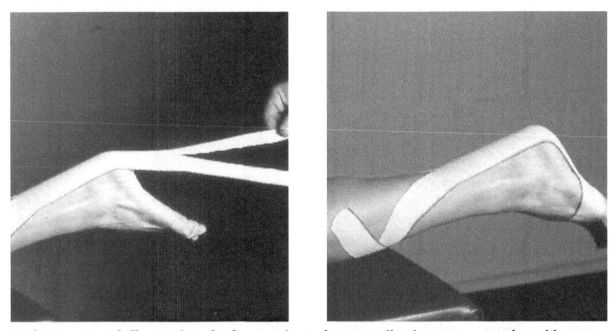

Technique A: Achilles tendon check rein. This technique will aid in preventing the ankle joint from excessive dorsiflexion. Using 3-in. elastic tape, cut a strip 15 in. to 20 in. in length, split both ends lengthwise approximately 5 in. to 7 in. With the ankle in plantar flexion, encircle the mid-portion of the lower leg with the split ends of the elastic tape. Pull the tape to full tension, crossing the heel and rear foot region. Encircle the mid-foot region with the other split ends of the elastic tape. Secure this technique with two anchors of 1½-in. adhesive tape.

Adjunct Padding Procedure: Achilles Tendon

These adjunct padding procedures can be used in conjunction with the basic technique presented.

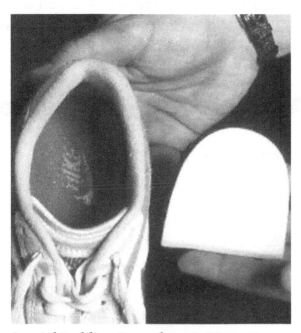 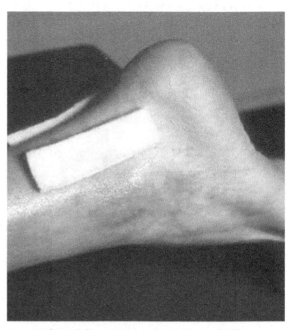

3

Special Padding Procedure A. Using ½-in. felt, cut a heel lift to be placed in the posterior aspect of the shoe. Place a similar felt heel lift in the shoe of the unaffected foot.

Special Padding Procedure B: Achilles tendon strips. To reduce pressure on the tendon, cut two strips of ½-in. felt, 1 in. x 3 in. Place one strip lateral and a second strip medial to the Achilles tendon. This will help reduce pressure on the Achilles tendon when the shoe is worn.

Wrapping Techniques for Support

During physical activity, supportive wraps are used to aid in muscle function and support and to reduce excessive range of motion. These applications are typically used in competition or practice. Spica wraps are traditionally employed at the hip and shoulder joints. Figure of eight wraps are placed over ankle, knee, elbow, wrist, and hand joints.

Ankle Wrap–Cohesive

Purpose:	To provide support to the ankle joint
Clinical Application:	Ankle sprains
Anatomical Structure:	Ankle joint
Anatomical Position:	Ankle in neutral position (90 degrees)
Supplies:	Cohesive tape
Pre-Wrapping Procedures:	With the ankle in neutral position, instruct the individual to contract the muscles of the foot, ankle, and lower leg

Wrapping Procedure: A continuous wrap is used in this preventive technique and consists of a figure of 8 and medial and lateral heel locks and finishes with a figure of 8.

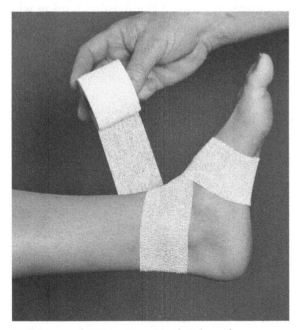

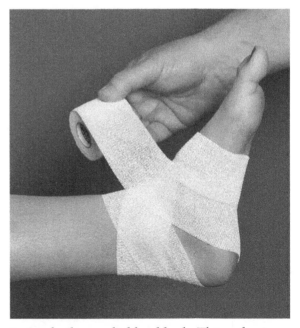

1. Figure of 8. Starting on the dorsal aspect of the foot, move medially down the inside of the foot, across the plantar portion, up the outside of the foot to the starting point. Continuation of the cohesive tape will proceed medially around the lower leg, crossing the Achilles tendon, returning to the origin of this figure of 8 technique.

2. Apply the medial heel lock. This cohesive tape continues across the medial malleolus, crosses the Achilles tendon, goes around the lateral aspect of the heel, angles underneath the foot, and moves up to the dorsum of the foot.

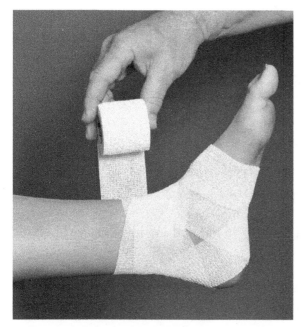

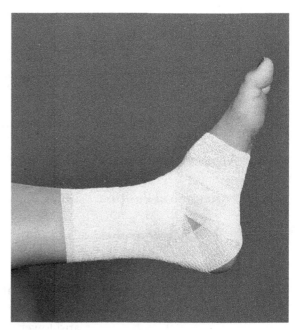

3. Continue the lateral heel lock across the lateral malleolus, cross the Achilles tendon, go around the medial aspect of the heel, angle underneath the foot, and move up to the dorsum of the foot.

4. Repeat Step 1 (figure of 8 wrap).

*Upon completion of the procedure, make sure you check for neatness and gaps, adequate support, along with proper function of the affected area. In certain situations, the individual might be asked to perform function tests to establish appropriate technique.

3

Ankle Wrap–Cloth

Purpose:	To provide support to the ankle joint
Clinical Application:	Ankle sprains
Anatomical Structure:	Ankle joint
Anatomical Position:	Ankle in neutral position (90 degrees)
Supplies:	2-in. cloth wrap (72 in. to 96 in.) and 1½-in. adhesive or elastic tape
Pre-Wrapping Procedures:	With the ankle in neutral position, apply the athletic sock. Instruct the individual to contract the muscles of the foot, ankle, and lower leg

Wrapping Procedure: A continuous wrap is used in this preventive technique and consists of a figure of eight and medial and lateral heel locks and finishes with a figure of 8.

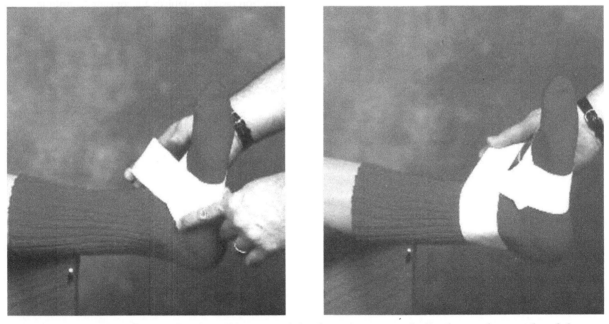

1. Figure of 8. Starting on the dorsal aspect of the foot, move medially down the inside of the foot, across the plantar portion, up the outside of the foot to the starting point. Continue the wrap medially around the lower leg, crossing the Achilles tendon, returning to the origin of this figure of 8 technique.

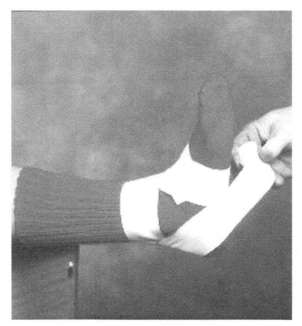

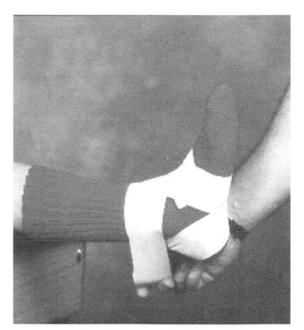

2. Apply the medial heel lock. This wrap continues across the medial malleolus, crosses the Achilles tendon, goes around the lateral aspect of the heel, angles underneath the foot, and moves up to the dorsum of the foot.

3. Continue the lateral heel lock wrap across the lateral malleolus, move across the Achilles tendon, go around the medial aspect of the heel, angle underneath the foot, and move up to the dorsum of the foot.

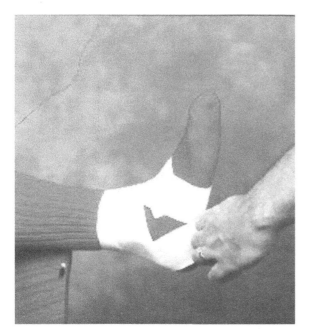

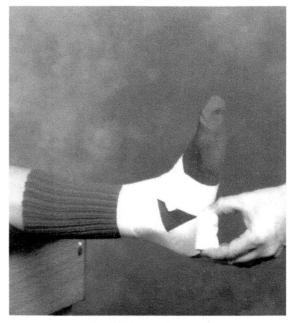

4. Repeat Step 1 (figure of 8 wrap).

3

3

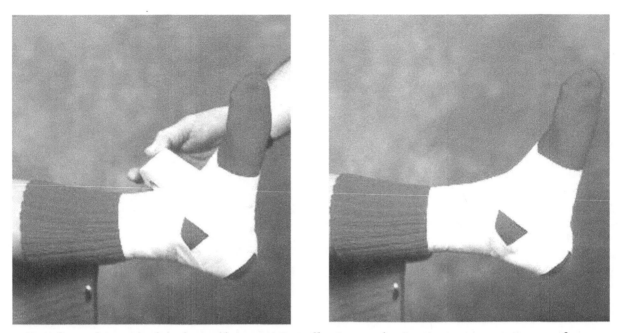

5. Reinforce this procedure by applying 1½-in. adhesive or elastic tape to construct extra figures of 8 and heel locks over the cloth wrap.

*Upon completion of the procedure, make sure you check for neatness and gaps, adequate support, along with proper function of the affected area. In certain situations, the individual might be asked to perform function tests to establish appropriate technique application.

Protective Devices

The use of protective devices is beneficial if they are properly selected, used in the appropriate setting, correctly fitted, and follow the guidelines of the specific sport. Consultation with a medical equipment specialist is highly encouraged! In some cases, a prescription from a licensed physician may result in insurance reimbursement. Listed below are various protective devices that are commercially available for use in sports and/or physical activity.

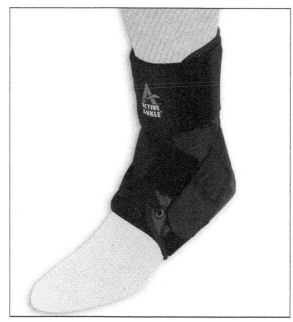

Active Ankle AS-1 Ankle Support

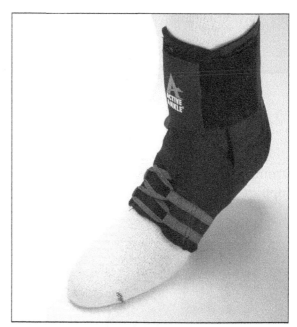

Active Ankle Excel Ankle Brace

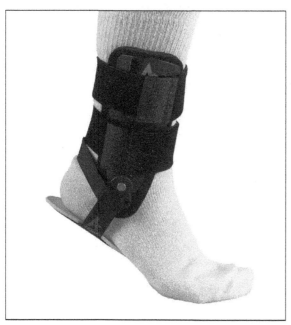

T1 Active Ankle Trainer's Model

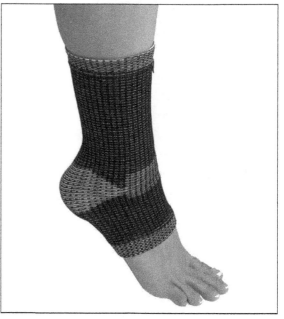

Stromgren Nano Flex Ankle

3

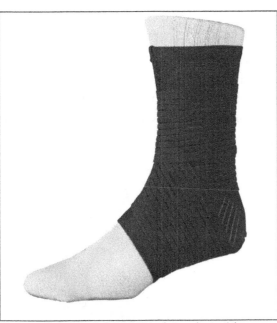

Stromgren Model 329 Heel-Lock Ankle Support

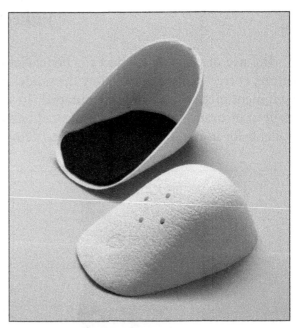

Cramer Padded Heel Cups

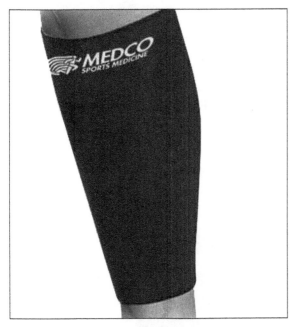

Medco Neoprene Calf Support

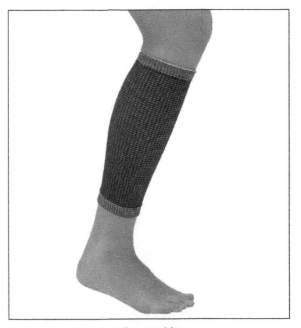

Stromgren Nano Flex Calf Support

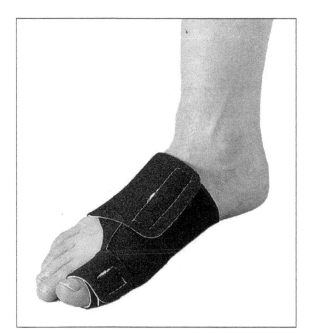

Rolyan Bunion Splint

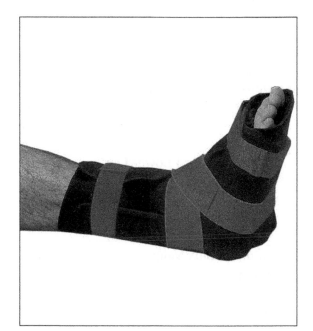

Rolyan Plantar Fasciitis Splint

3

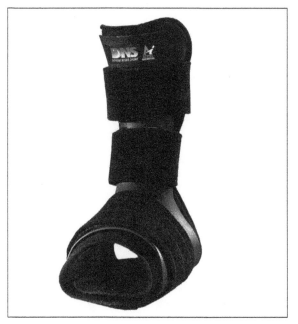

Cramer Dorsal Night Splint

Listed below are various protective devices available to use in sport. Because a variety of protective devices are available, a qualified physician or qualified health care professional and medical equipment specialist can determine whether the individual is best suited for an off-the-shelf or custom brace.
- Achilles tendon strap
- Boots (hockey, ski, wrestling)
- Orthotics (soft, semirigid, rigid)
- Shin guards
- Turf toe brace

Musculoskeletal Disorders

The following is a list of common musculoskeletal disorders of the foot, ankle, and lower leg. For definitions of these terms, the authors encourage the learner to consult these medical references: *Taber's Medical Dictionary, Stedman's Medical Dictionary for the Health Professions and Nursing,* and/or *Signs and Symptoms of Athletic Injuries* (listed in Appendix B).

3

Foot, Ankle, and Lower Leg

Achilles tendinitis/tendinosis
Ankle sprain
Apophysitis calcaneus
Arch sprain
Bunion (Hallux Valgus)
Bunionette
Bursitis
Corn
Great toe sprain
Hallux rigidus
Hallux varus
Hammer toe
Heel spur
Interdigital neuroma
Mallet toe
Morton's neuroma
Plantar aponeurosis (Plantar fasciitis)
Plantar neuroma
Retrocalcaneal achilles bursitis
Sesamoiditis
Shin splints
Stone bruise
Talotibial exostosis
Tarsal tunnel syndrome
Tendinitis/tenosynovitis

4 Knee, Thigh, and Hip

Educational Objectives

Upon completing this chapter, the reader will be able to do the following:
- Identify anatomical landmarks critical for correct taping procedures
- Describe the purpose for the applications of adhesive and elastic tape
- Select the proper supplies and specialty items used for taping
- Explain the steps in preparing the body for taping, wrapping, or protective device
- Describe and demonstrate the purposes, clinical applications, anatomical structures, supplies needed, and pre-taping and taping procedures for anatomical areas
- Identify the proper use and application of protective devices for the knee, thigh, and hip

Introduction

Techniques for lower extremities can be meaningful when injuries occur to the knee, thigh, and hip. Therefore, a basic foundation in understanding the area is important for injury care. This chapter will highlight the terminology, taping techniques, wrapping techniques, protective devices, and musculoskeletal disorders associated with the knee, thigh, and hip.

Terminology

Flexion. Movement around a transverse axis in an anterior–posterior plane with the angle between the anterior aspects of the displaced parts becoming smaller, as in bending the forearm toward the arm at the elbow joint; the act of drawing a body segment away from a straight line with its proximally conjoined body segment or toward smallest acute angle of that joint.

Extension. The reverse movement during which the angle between the anterior aspects of the displaced parts is increased, as in moving the forearm away from the upper arm; the act of drawing a body segment toward a straight line position with its proximally conjoined body segment or away from the body joint.

Abduction. Movement away from the median plane around an anterior–posterior axis with the angle between the displaced parts becoming greater, as in lifting the arm sideward away from the body; the act of drawing a body segment away from the median line of the body.

Adduction. Movement toward the median plane around an anterior–posterior axis with the angle between the displaced parts becoming lesser, as in bringing the arm sideward against the body; the act of drawing a body segment toward the median line of the body.

Rotation. Movement around a longitudinal axis that passes through a joint, as in turning the palm of the hand up or down with the arm abducted.

Valgus. Position of a body part that is bent outward.

Varus. Position of a body part that is bent inward.

Quadriceps. The muscle group in the anterior thigh consisting of the rectus femoris, vastus medialis, vastus intermedius, and vastus lateralis.

Hamstrings. A muscle group in the posterior thigh consisting of the semitendinosus, semimembranosus, and biceps femoris.

Popliteal space. Area behind the knee joint.

Anterior cruciate ligament (ACL). A ligament crossing through the knee joint that attaches from the anterior tibia to the posterior femur. It limits anterior movement of the tibia from the femur, as well as rotation of the tibia.

Knee, Thigh, and Hip

4

Taping Techniques and Protective Devices

Developing a thorough knowledge regarding the fundamentals of the application of taping/wrapping procedures is imperative. Review Chapter 1 before applying any technique.

Proper Assessment of Injury

Before applying a preventive technique (tape, wrap, and/or device), a qualified physician or qualified health care professional should complete a proper injury evaluation. Following injury evaluation, the professional can then recommend proper taping techniques. This ensures that proper taping techniques are applied for support and stabilization. Also, developing a thorough knowledge of taping application fundamentals is imperative.

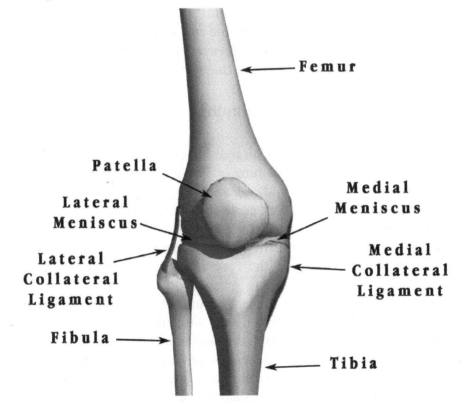

Figure 4.1. Bony anatomy of the knee

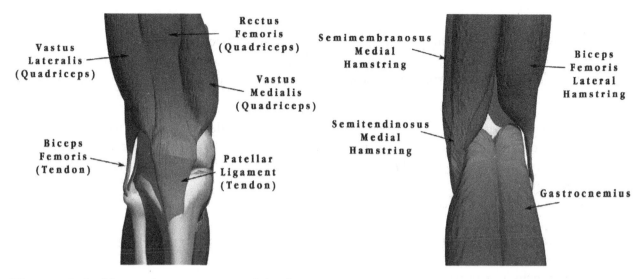

Figure 4.2. Muscular anatomy of the knee

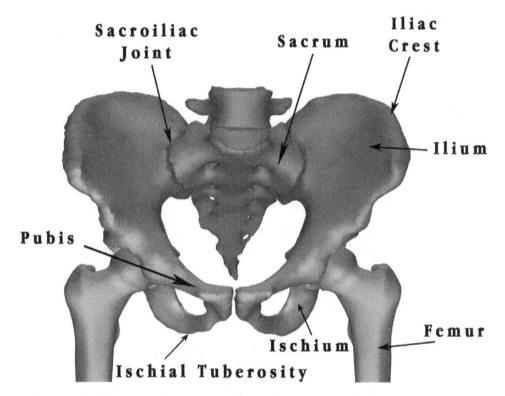

4

Figure 4.3. Bony anatomy of the hip and pelvis

Purpose and Application of Adhesive and Elastic Tape

The primary purpose for tape application is to provide additional support and stability for the affected body part. Through proper application, taping techniques can be applied to shorten the muscle's angle of pull; to decrease joint range of motion; to secure pads, bandages, and protective devices; and to apply compression to reduce swelling.

Medical Supplies and Specialty Items

Purchasing supplies depends on budget, philosophy of medical staff regarding taping techniques, and occurrence of injury. Review Chapter 1 before applying any technique.

Specific Rules on Taping, Wrapping, and/or Protective Device

If you apply supportive techniques to an individual, you should be aware of specific rules governing tape application in that particular sport or physical activity. Your application must fall within the guidelines established for each sport by appropriate governing bodies.

Special Techniques: Adjunct Taping Procedures

The taping techniques presented are the fundamental procedures. Adjunct techniques will be shown to provide additional support; however, you should still follow the fundamental procedures. Variations can be achieved by adapting these techniques to a particular injury situation. Always give special consideration to

- purpose of the taping procedure
- clinical application
- correct anatomical position
- supply selection
- tape/wrap technique or protective device

Preparation of Body Part for Taping

In preparing the body for tape application, consider these six items:

1. removal of hair (optional)
2. clean the area
3. special considerations
4. spray adherent (optional)
5. skin lubricants
6. underwrap or cohesive tape

Proper Body Positioning

Before beginning a taping procedure, select a comfortable table height and ask the individual to assume an anatomically correct and comfortable position.

- Neutral Position of Knee: The knee should be in slight flexion (10 to 15 degrees).
- Neutral Position of Hip Joint: The hip and knee joint should be placed in slight flexion.

When applying a technique, learn to stand at a comfortable and stationary position and place the body part to be taped at your elbow height.

Taping Techniques

The taping techniques presented are the fundamental procedures. A strong knowledge of anatomy, physiology, and biomechanics is essential. Developing a thorough knowledge regarding the fundamentals about the application of taping/wrapping procedures is imperative. Review Chapter 1 before applying any technique.

Collateral Knee

Purpose:	To provide support and stability to the collateral ligaments of the knee
Clinical Application:	Sprains
Anatomical Structure:	Knee joint
Anatomical Position:	Knee joint in slight flexion (10 to 15 degrees)
Supplies:	1½-in. adhesive tape, 3-in. elastic tape, and gauze with lubricant (heel and lace pad)

4

Pre-Taping Procedure:

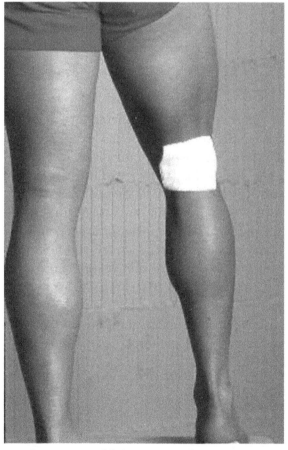

Apply gauze and lubricant to the posterior aspect (popliteal space) of the knee joint

Taping Procedure:

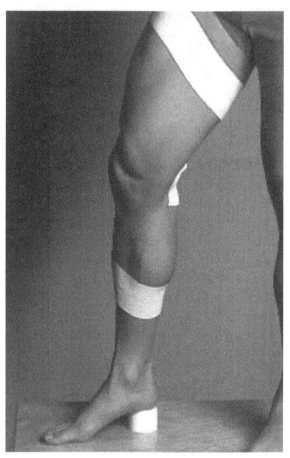

1. Apply two anchor strips of 3-in. elastic tape to the extremity. Place the proximal anchor strip at the mid-thigh or higher. Apply the distal anchor at the mid-gastrocnemius region or lower. Attach all collateral strips on these two anchors.

4

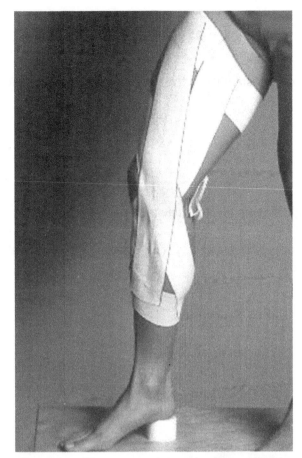

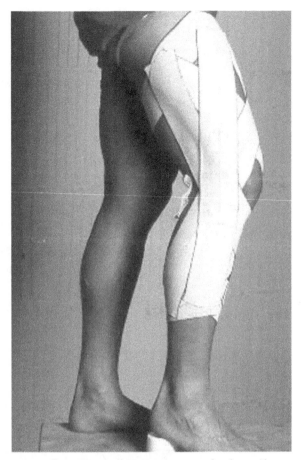

2. Apply collateral X pattern to the medial side of the knee. Using 3-in. elastic tape, start on the lateral aspect of the distal anchor, come below the patella, cross the medial joint line, and attach to the posteromedial aspect of the proximal anchor. Begin the second strip on the posterior aspect of the distal anchor, cross the medial joint line, and attach to the anterior portion of the proximal anchor. Apply a third strip vertically on the medial side. Begin this support strip on the distal anchor, cross the joint line, and attach to the proximal anchor.

3. Apply collateral X pattern to the lateral side of the knee. Using 3-in. elastic tape, start on the medial aspect of the distal anchor, come below the patella, cross the lateral joint line, and attach to the posterolateral aspect of the proximal anchor. Begin the second strip on the posterior aspect of the distal anchor, cross the lateral joint line, and attach to the anterior portion of the proximal anchor. Apply a third strip vertically on the lateral side. Begin this support strip on the distal anchor, cross the joint line, and attach to the proximal anchor.

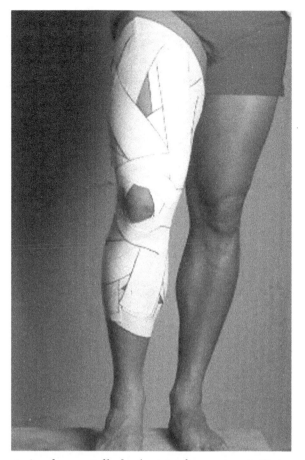

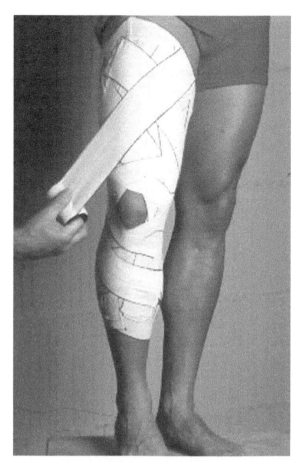

4. Apply a patella lock strip for support. Cut a strip of 3-in. elastic tape, 15 in. to 20 in. in length. Center this patella lock strip over the popliteal fossa. Split each end approximately 4 in. to 6 in. Cover the joint line and place the medial split ends inferior and superior to the patella. Apply the lateral split ends in the same manner. The four split ends should form a diamond shape near the patella.

5. Apply two spiral strips to protect the popliteal fossa and to assist in preventing hyperextension. Using 3-in. elastic tape, begin on the anterior portion of the proximal anchor, and moving medially, spiral posteriorly, crossing the popliteal fossa, and complete the strip on the anterior portion of the distal anchor. Repeat this sequence a second time, applying the tape laterally.

4

4

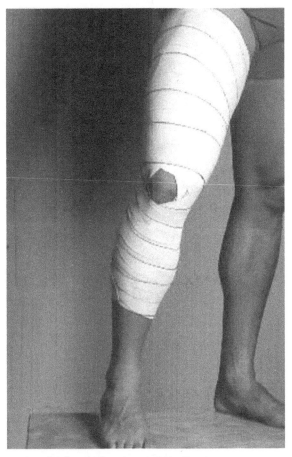

6. Apply final closure strips. Begin
proximally and work distally. From the
upper anchor, apply individual circular strips
around the extremity to cover tape ends.
Overlap the tape approximately one half of
its width on each strip. Secure the elastic tape
ends with anchors of 1½-in. adhesive tape.

*Upon completion of the procedure, make sure you
check for neatness and gaps, adequate support, along
with proper function of the affected area. In certain
situations, the individual might be asked to perform
function tests to establish appropriate technique
application.

Adjunct Taping Procedure: Collateral Knee

This adjunct taping procedure can be used in conjunction with the basic technique presented.

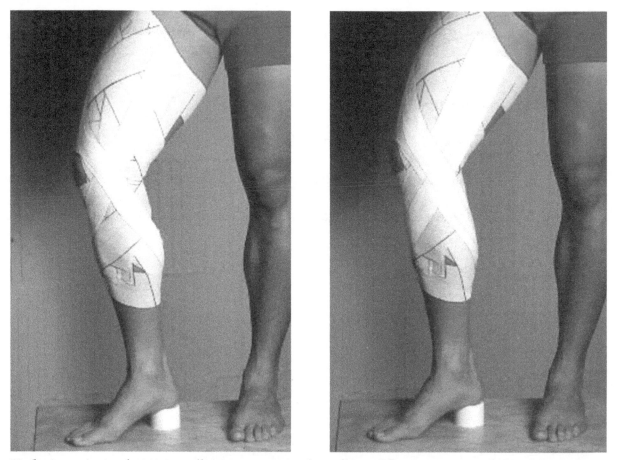

4

Technique A. Apply 1½-in. adhesive tape over the collateral X patterns to provide additional support.

Hyperextended Knee

Purpose:	To assist in prevention of knee joint hyperextension
Clinical Application:	Hyperextension sprain
Anatomical Structure:	Knee joint
Anatomical Position:	Knee joint placed in slight flexion
Supplies:	1½-in. adhesive tape, 3-in. elastic tape, and gauze with lubricant
Pre-Taping Procedures:	Apply the gauze with lubricant to the popliteal fossa of the knee joint

4

Taping Procedure:

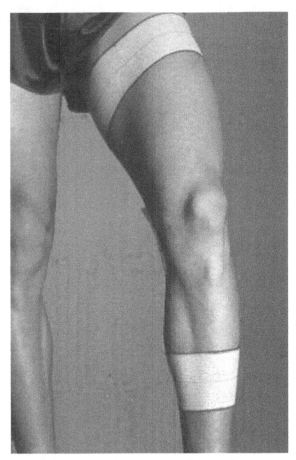

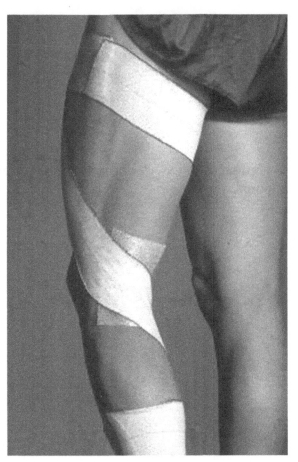

1. Apply two anchor strips of 3-in. elastic tape to the extremity. Place the proximal anchor strip at the mid-thigh or higher. Apply the distal anchor at the mid-gastrocnemius region or lower.

2. Using 3-in. elastic tape, begin on the anterior portion of the distal anchor, move laterally and spiral posteriorly, crossing the popliteal fossa, and complete the strip on the anterior portion of the proximal anchor.

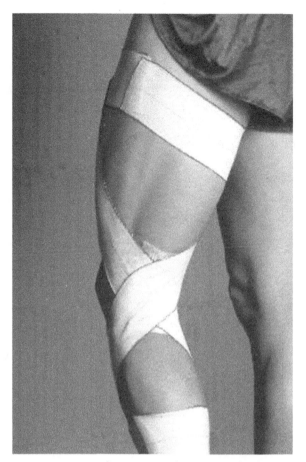

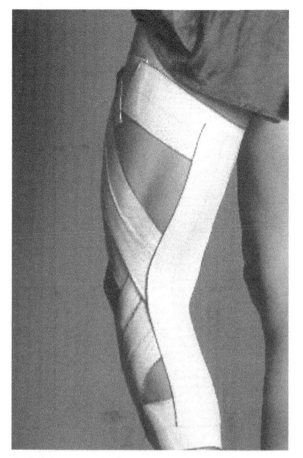

3. Using 3-in. elastic tape, begin on the anterior portion of the proximal anchor, and moving medially, spiral posteriorly, crossing the popliteal fossa, and complete this strip on the anterior portion of the distal anchor.

4. Apply a vertical strip starting on the proximal anchor, cross the popliteal fossa, and end on the distal anchor. Repeat steps 2, 3, and 4 a second time for additional support. Exercise **caution** when encircling the lower leg to avoid undue pressure on the musculature.

4

4

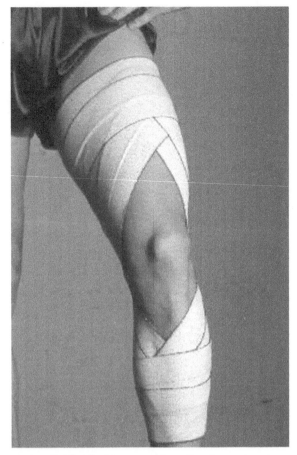

5. Apply final closure strips. Begin proximally and work distally. From the upper anchor, apply individual circular strips around the extremity to cover tape ends. Make sure you overlap the tape approximately one half of its width on each strip. Optional: secure the elastic tape ends with anchors of 1½-in. adhesive tape.

*Upon completion of the procedure, make sure you check for neatness and gaps, adequate support, along with proper function of the affected area. In certain situations, the individual might be asked to perform function tests to establish appropriate technique application.

Adjunct Taping Procedures: Hyperextended Knee

This adjunct taping procedure can be used in conjunction with the basic technique presented.

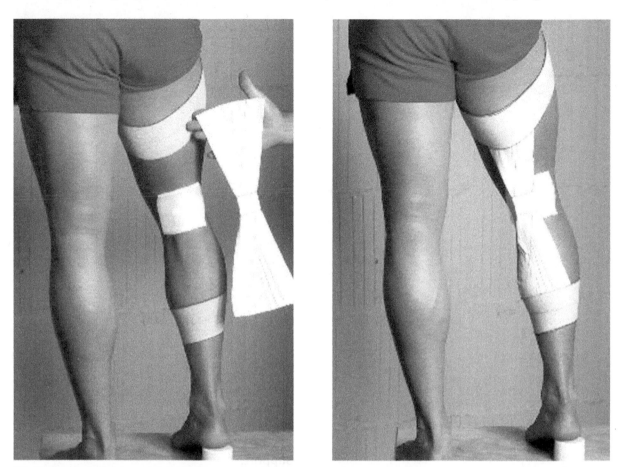

Technique A. Using either adhesive or elastic tape, construct a five- to seven-strip butterfly (hour glass) pattern that will extend from the proximal to the distal anchors. Prior to application, place a strip of tape around the mid-portion of this support pattern. Place the support on the proximal anchor, pull downward, and attach to the distal anchor. Secure this technique with strips of elastic tape over the proximal and distal anchor. This technique should help restrict hyperextension of the knee joint.

4

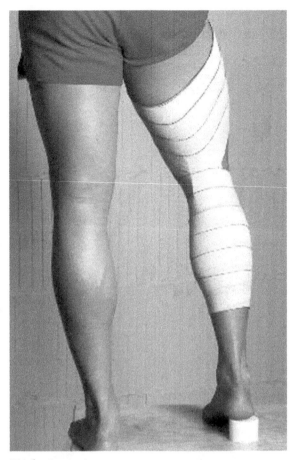

Technique A.

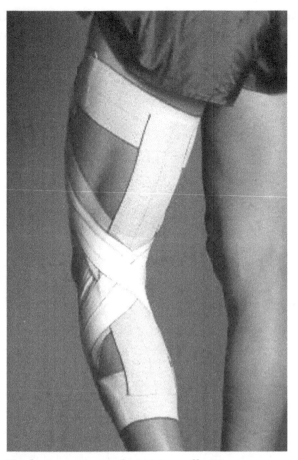

Technique B. Apply 1½-in. adhesive tape over the spiral strips to provide additional support.

Anterior Cruciate

Purpose:	To enhance support and stability to the anterior cruciate ligament of the knee
Clinical Application:	Sprain to anterior cruciate ligament
Anatomical Structure:	Knee
Anatomical Position:	Knee and hip joints should be positioned in slight flexion
Supplies:	1½-in. adhesive tape, 3-in. elastic tape, and gauze with lubricant

4

Pre-Taping Procedure:

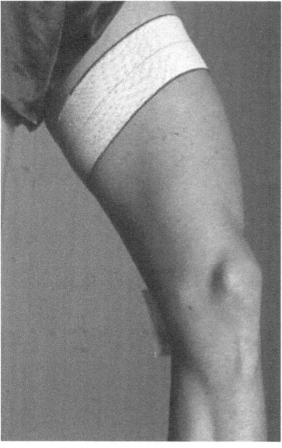

With the knee and hip joints in slight flexion, apply the gauze with lubricant to the posterior aspect of the knee joint. Also apply an anchor strip of 3-in. elastic tape around the upper third of the thigh. *Comment:* In this pre-taping procedure, do not compress the popliteal fossa.

Taping Procedure:

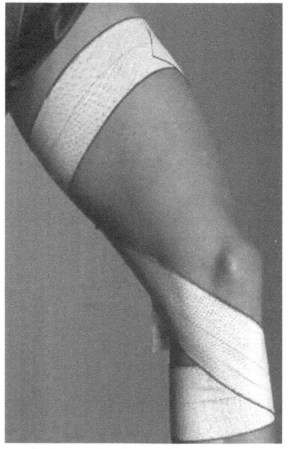

1. Using 3-in. elastic tape, begin on the lower lateral aspect of the leg, approximately 1 in. below the patella. Encircle the lower leg, moving anteriorly and then medially, continuing to the posterior aspect, and returning to the lateral side. Angle the tape below the patella, cross the medial joint line and popliteal fossa, and spiral up to anchor on the anterior portion of the upper thigh.

4

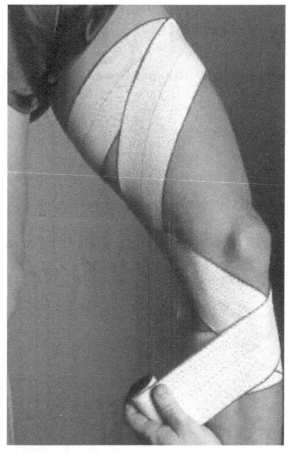

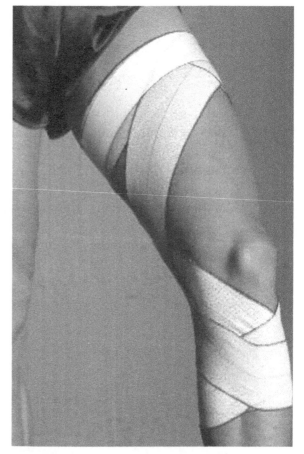

2. Begin the next strip of 3-in. elastic tape on the anterior aspect of the proximal anchor and cross medial portion of the thigh, covering the popliteal fossa, encircling the lower leg, and crossing the popliteal fossa again. Finish by spiraling up to anchor on the anterior aspect of the thigh.

3. Repeat Step 2. Secure this technique by applying 1½-in. adhesive tape over the anchor on the thigh.

*Upon completion of the procedure, make sure you check for neatness and gaps, adequate support, along with proper function of the affected area. In certain situations, the individual might be asked to perform function tests to establish appropriate technique application.

Patella Tendon

Purpose:	To reduce stress on the patella tendon
Clinical Application:	Patella tendon strain and tendinitis
Anatomical Structure:	Patella tendon
Anatomical Position:	Knee joint slightly flexed and muscles of lower leg relaxed
Supplies:	1-in. adhesive or elastic tape

Taping Procedure:

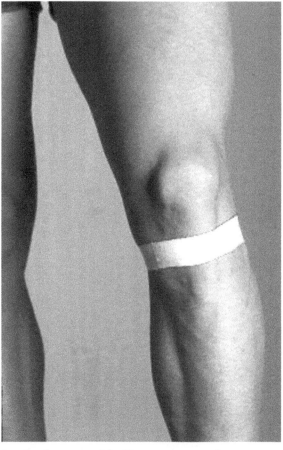

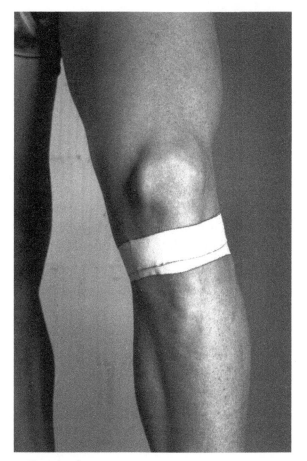

1. Apply tape with direct pressure between the distal end of the patella and superior aspect of the tibia tuberosity. Encircle the lower leg starting on the lateral side, move anteriorly and then to the medial side, continue to the posterior aspect, and return to the lateral side.

2. Repeat Step 1.

*Upon completion of the procedure, make sure you check for neatness and gaps, adequate support, along with proper function of the affected area. In certain situations, the individual might be asked to perform function tests to establish appropriate technique application.

Adjunct Taping Procedure: Patella Tendon Taping

4

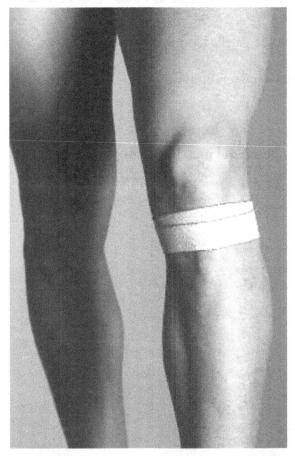

Technique A. In conjunction with the basic procedure, use 1-in. or 2-in. elastic tape in a continuous procedure for additional support.

Hip Pointer

Purpose: To provide support and protection to the contused tissue of the iliac crest

Clinical Application: Contusions and strains

Anatomical Structure: Iliac crest

Anatomical Position: Standing with slight lateral flexion of the waist to the affected side

Supplies: 1½-in. adhesive tape, 3-in. elastic tape, ½-in. foam pad, and 6-in. extra long elastic wrap

Pre-Taping Procedures: Cut a foam pad that will cover the affected area. In certain situations, construct a doughnut pad that will relieve pressure on the affected area.

4

Taping Procedure:

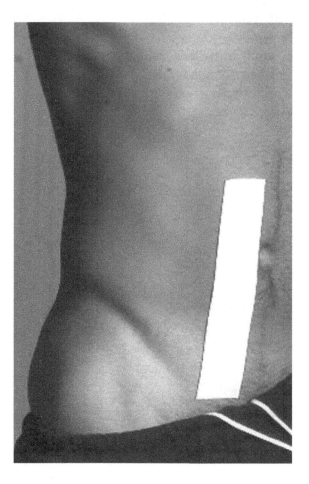

1. Apply two vertical anchor strips approximately 4 in. to 6 in. anteriorly and posteriorly to the affected area.

4

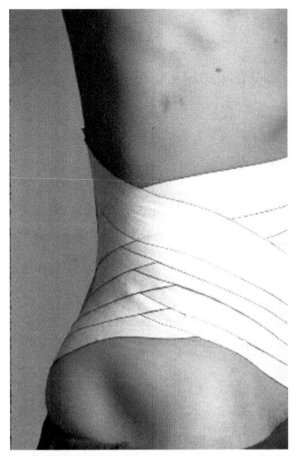

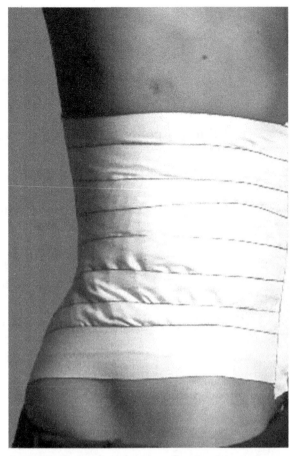

2. Apply the X pattern technique, overlapping by one half, beginning at the anterior aspect of the anchors, and moving posteriorly until the entire crest of the hip is covered.

3. Apply horizontal strips, beginning on the superior anchor, and moving inferiorly, overlap by one half until the entire area is covered.

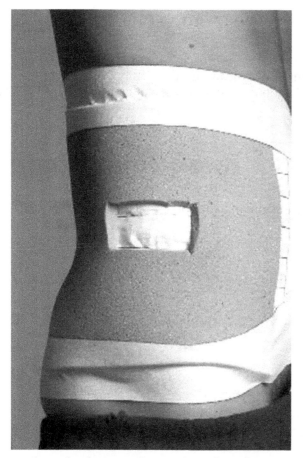

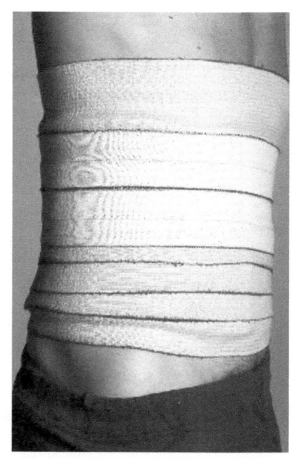

4. Place the foam pad over the affected area. This pad is held in place with two strips of adhesive tape.

*Upon completion of the procedure, make sure you check for neatness and gaps, adequate support, along with proper function of the affected area. In certain situations, the individual might be asked to perform function tests to establish appropriate technique application.

5. Have the individual inhale to expand the thorax when applying the elastic wrap. Then apply a strip of elastic tape over the wrap to secure the ends.

Adjunct Taping Procedure: Hip Pointer

   This adjunct taping procedure can be used in conjunction with the basic technique presented. **Technique A.** Under certain situations, the application of this hip flexor wrap is preferred. This wrap will encircle the complete thigh and waist region of the body. (Refer to Hip Flexor Wrap.)

Wrapping Techniques for Support

During physical activity, supportive wraps are used to aid in muscle function and support and to reduce excessive range of motion. These applications are typically used in competition or practice. Spica wraps are traditionally employed at the hip and shoulder joints. Figure of eight wraps are placed over ankle, knee, elbow, wrist, and hand joints.

Knee Joint Wrap

Purpose:	To provide compression and support to the knee joint
Clinical Application:	Sprains to the knee joint
Anatomical Structure:	Knee joint
Anatomical Position:	Knee joint placed in slight flexion, through a heel lift under the heel
Supplies:	4-in. double length elastic wrap and 1½-in. adhesive tape
Pre-Wrapping Procedure:	The individual should stand with the affected knee in slight flexion. Instruct the individual to contract the muscles around the knee joint.

Wrapping Procedures:

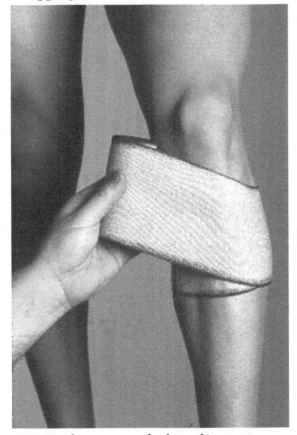

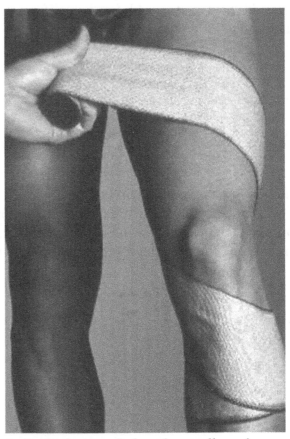

1. Begin the wrap on the lateral/posterior aspect of the lower leg. Encircle the lower leg, moving medially to laterally.

2. Angle the wrap below the patella and cross the medial joint line. Cover the posterior and lateral aspects of the thigh.

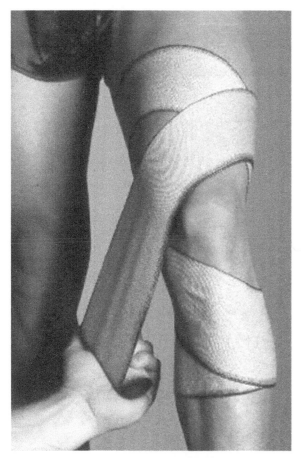

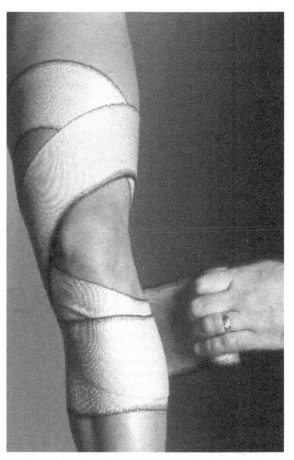

3. Encircle the thigh, moving medially to laterally. Angle the wrap downward, staying above the patella and crossing the medial joint line.

4. Cross the popliteal space and encircle the lower leg.

4

4

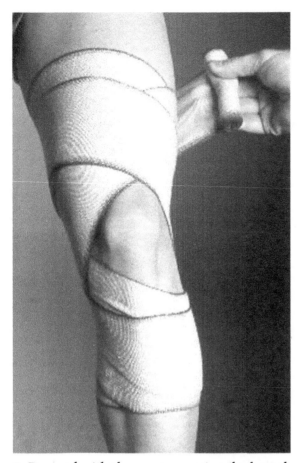

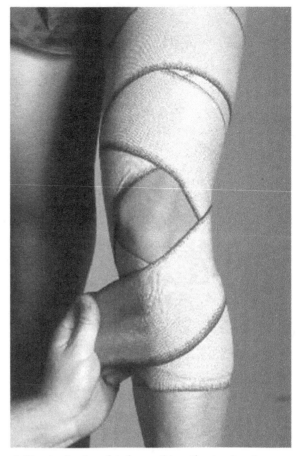

5. Proceed with the wrap, crossing the lateral joint line and angling above the patella.

6. Encircle the thigh, and on the posterior aspect, angle across the lateral joint line of the knee, staying below the patella. This configuration should resemble a diamond shape around the patella and cover from mid-thigh to the gastrocnemius belly.

Adjunct Taping Procedures: Knee Wrap

This adjunct taping procedure can be used in conjunction with the basic technique presented.

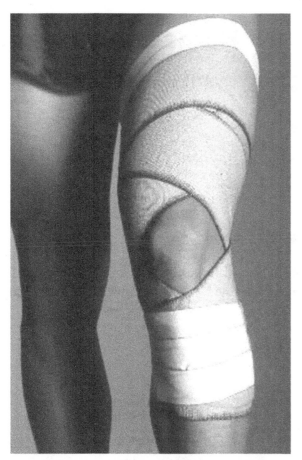

7. To secure this wrap, apply 1½-in. adhesive tape to the loose end of the wrap.

*Upon completion of the procedure, make sure you check for neatness and gaps, adequate support, along with proper function of the affected area. In certain situations, the individual might be asked to perform function tests to establish appropriate technique application.

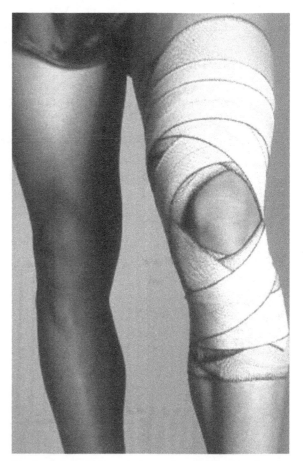

Technique A. In conjunction with the elastic wrap, you can use 2-in. or wider elastic tape in a continuous method.

4

Hamstring Wrap

Purpose:	To provide support to the hamstring muscle group
Clinical Application:	Strain to hamstring muscles
Anatomical Structure:	Posterior aspect of the thigh
Anatomical Position:	In standing position, affected extremity is in hip extension
Supplies:	1½-in. adhesive tape and 6-in. elastic wrap
Pre-Wrapping Procedure:	The individual should stand with the affected extremity placed in hip extension and the individual should contract the hamstring muscles

4

Wrapping Procedures:

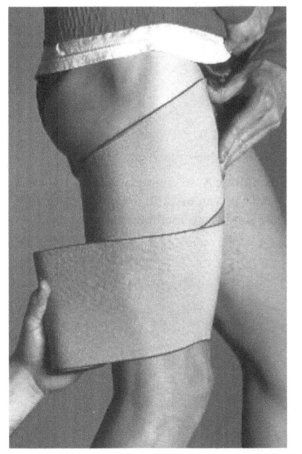 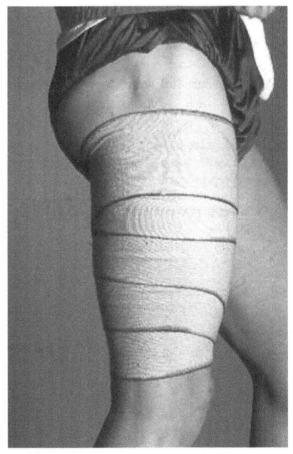

1. Begin the wrap at the proximal end of the thigh. Angle diagonally to the distal aspect of the hamstrings. At this point, begin an upward spiral supportive procedure with the wrap. Overlap each layer by one half of its width, ending at the proximal end of the thigh.

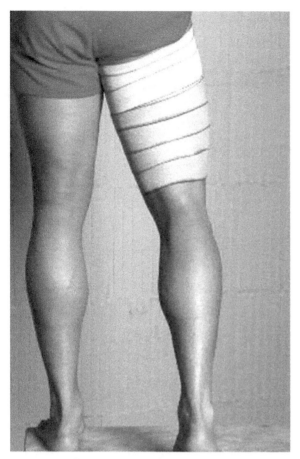

2. Secure the wrap in place by applying an anchor strip of 1½-in. adhesive tape.

*Upon completion of the procedure, make sure you check for neatness and gaps, adequate support, along with proper function of the affected area. In certain situations, the individual might be asked to perform function tests to establish appropriate technique application.

Adjunct Taping Procedures: Hamstring Wrap

This adjunct taping procedure can be used in conjunction with the basic technique presented.

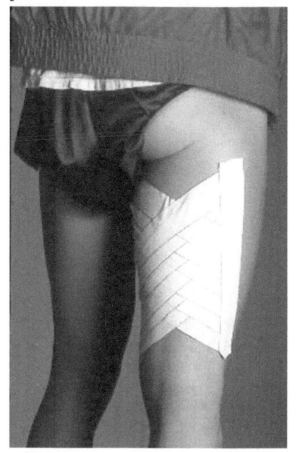

Technique A: The X pattern technique.
Apply the wrap over this technique for additional support. Apply two vertical anchor strips approximately 4 in. to 6 in. anteriorly and posteriorly to the affected area. Overlap by one half, beginning at the anterior aspect of the anchors and moving posteriorly until the entire area is covered.

4

4

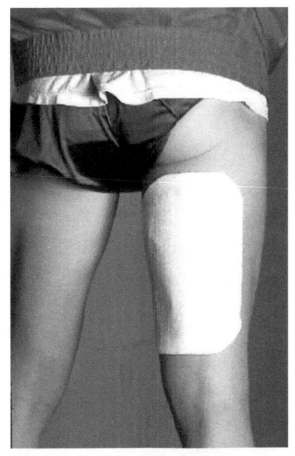

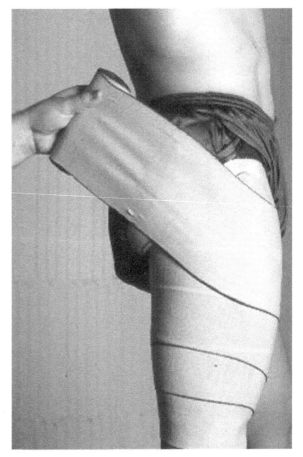

Technique B: Felt pad. Apply a 3-in. x 5-in. (or larger) felt pad over the affected area. Using ½-in. felt, apply the wrap over this technique for additional support and compression.

Technique C: Hip extension wrap. Using a 6-in. double length elastic wrap, apply a hip spica wrap, encircling the complete thigh and waist region of the body.

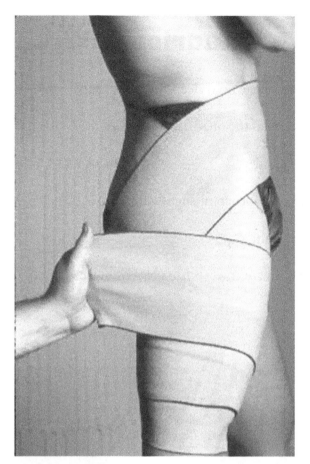 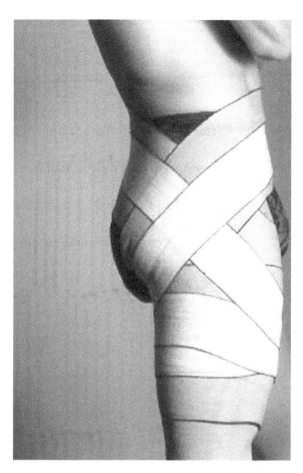

Technique C.

4

Quadriceps Wrap

Purpose:	To provide support for the quadriceps muscle group
Clinical Application:	Strain and contusions to the quadriceps muscles
Anatomical Structure:	Thigh
Anatomical Position:	Standing with hip and knee joint slightly flexed
Supplies:	1½-in. adhesive tape and 6-in. elastic wrap
Pre-Wrapping Procedure:	The individual should contract the quadriceps muscle group

4

Wrapping Procedures:

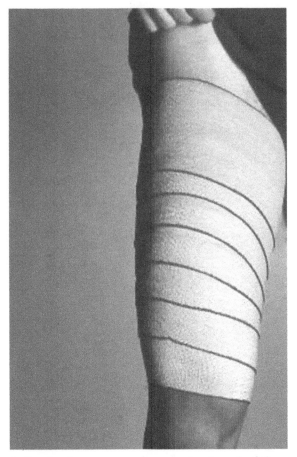

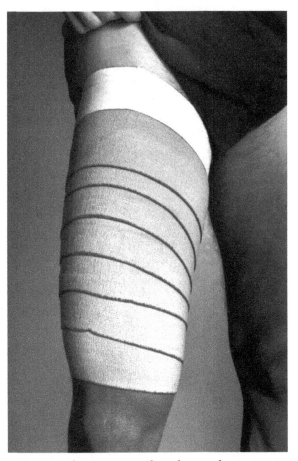

1. Begin the wrap at the proximal end of the thigh. Angle diagonally to the distal aspect of the quadriceps. At this point, begin an upward spiral supportive procedure with the wrap. Overlap each layer by one half of its width, ending at the proximal end of the thigh.

2. Secure the wrap in place by applying an anchor strip of 1½-in. adhesive tape.

*Upon completion of the procedure, make sure you check for neatness and gaps, adequate support, along with proper function of the affected area. In certain situations, the individual might be asked to perform function tests to establish appropriate technique application.

Adjunct Taping Procedures: Quadriceps Wrap
   These adjunct taping procedures can be used in conjunction with the basic technique presented.

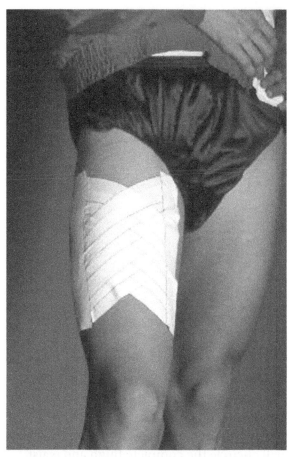

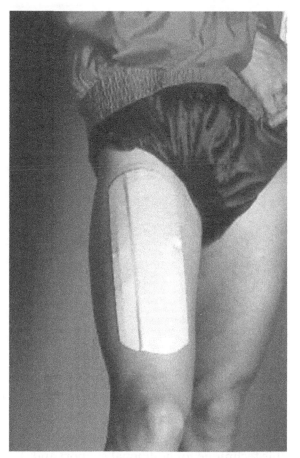

4

Technique A: The X pattern technique.
Apply the wrap over this technique for
additional support.

Technique B: Adhesive felt. Apply adhesive
felt over the affected area of the anterior
thigh.

4

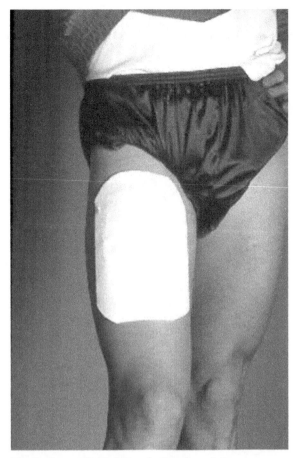

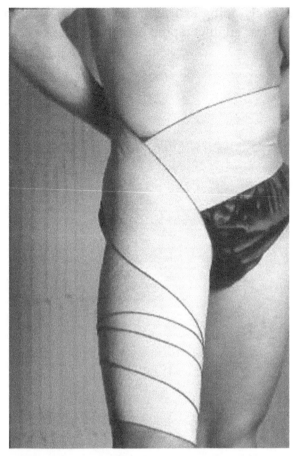

Technique C: Felt pad. Apply a 3-in. x 5-in. (or larger) felt pad (½ in. thick) over the affected area. Apply the wrap over this technique for additional support and compression.

Technique D: Thigh/hip flexion wrap. Under certain situations, the application of this hip flexor wrap is preferred. This wrap will encircle the complete thigh and waist region of the body.

Hip Flexor Wrap

Purpose:	To provide support to the hip flexor
Clinical Application:	Strain to the hip flexors
Anatomical Structure:	Hip and thigh
Anatomical Position:	The individual should stand with the affected extremity placed in hip flexion and the foot in slight internal rotation. The elastic wrap is continually applied in a hip spica method, abducting the thigh in the process.
Supplies:	6-in. extra long elastic wrap and 1½-in. adhesive tape
Pre-Wrapping Procedure:	The individual should contract the muscles around the hip joint

4

Wrapping Procedures:

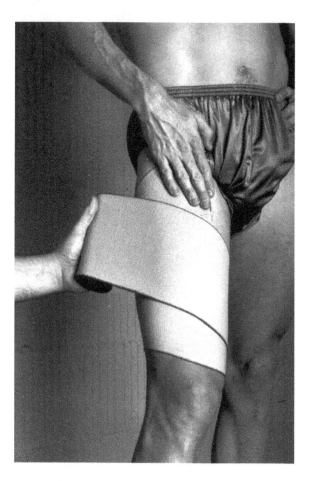

1. Begin the wrap at the proximal end of the thigh. From the anterior surface, angle diagonally to the distal lateral aspect of the quadriceps. Above the knee, begin an upward spiral supportive procedure with the wrap. Overlap each layer by one half of its width.

4

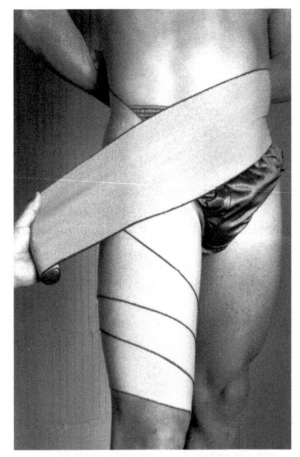 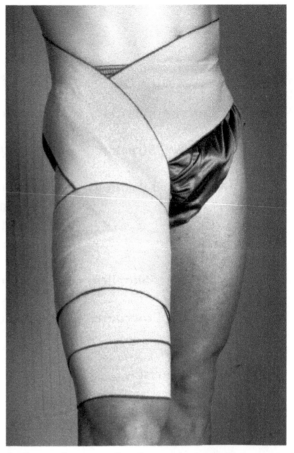

2. At the proximal end of the thigh, continue the wrap around the waist, pulling to the lateral and posterior aspect.

3. Once the waist has been encircled, continue the wrap around the thigh two to three times.

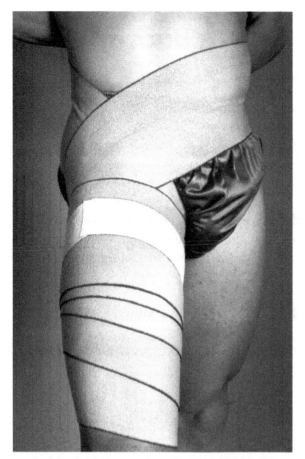

4. At this point, continue the wrap around the waist. This upward and outward pull should assist in hip flexion and limit hip extension. End the wrap on the thigh. Secure the wrap in place by applying an anchor strip of 1½-in. adhesive tape.

*Upon completion of the procedure, make sure you check for neatness and gaps, adequate support, along with proper function of the affected area. In certain situations, the individual might be asked to perform function tests to establish appropriate technique application.

Adjunct Taping Procedure: Hip Flexor Wrap

This adjunct taping procedure can be used in conjunction with the basic technique presented.

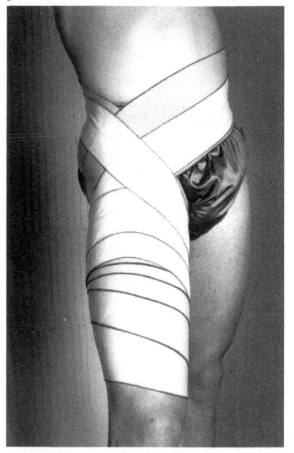

Technique A. Using 3-in. elastic tape, apply the tape over the wrap following the same pattern.

Hip Adductor Wrap

VIDEO

Purpose:	To provide support to the hip adductors
Clinical Application:	Strain to the hip adductors
Anatomical Structure:	Hip and thigh
Anatomical Position:	Individual should stand with the affected extremity placed in hip flexion and the foot in slight internal rotation. Continually apply the elastic wrap in a hip spica method, adducting the thigh in the process.
Supplies:	6-in. extra long elastic wrap and 1½-in. adhesive tape
Pre-Wrapping Procedure:	The individual should contract the muscles around the hip joint

Wrapping Procedures:

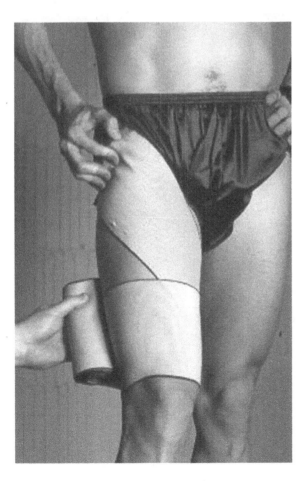

1. Begin the wrap at the proximal end of the thigh. From the anterior surface, angle diagonally to the distal medial aspect of the quadriceps. Above the knee, begin an upward spiral supportive procedure with the wrap. Overlap each layer by one half of its width.

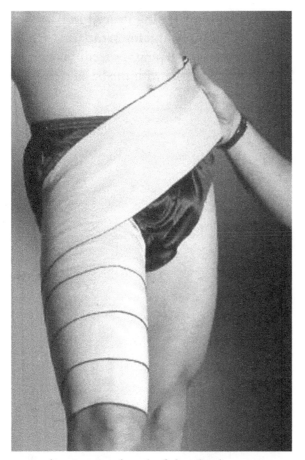

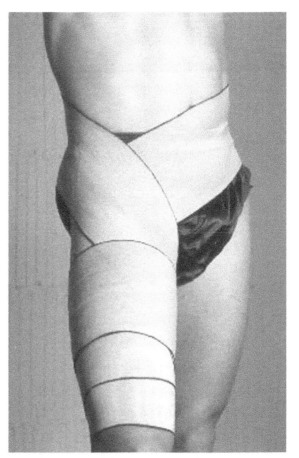

2. At the proximal end of the thigh, continue the wrap around the waist, pull across the abdomen to the lateral aspect and then to the posterior aspect. This upward and anterior pull should assist in hip adduction and limit hip abduction.

3. Once the waist has been encircled, continue the wrap downward and around the quadriceps muscle group two to three times.

4

4

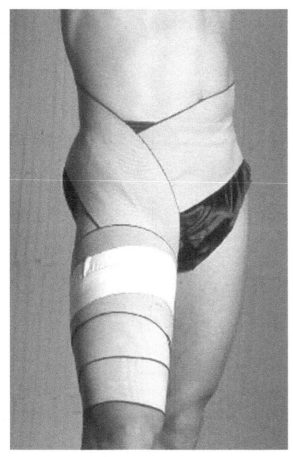

4. At this point, pull the wrap around the waist, crossing the abdomen, lateral, and posterior aspects. End the wrap on the thigh. Secure the wrap in place by applying an anchor strip of 1½-in. adhesive tape.

*Upon completion of the procedure, make sure you check for neatness and gaps, adequate support, along with proper function of the affected area. In certain situations, the individual might be asked to perform function tests to establish appropriate technique application.

Adjunct Taping Procedure: Hip Adductor Wrap

This adjunct taping procedure can be used in conjunction with the basic technique presented.

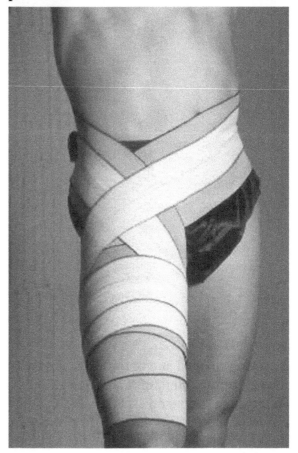

Technique A. Using 3-in. elastic tape, apply the tape over the wrap following the same pattern.

Protective Devices

The use of protective devices is beneficial if they are properly selected, used in the appropriate setting, correctly fitted, and follow the guidelines of the specific sport. Consultation with a medical equipment specialist is highly encouraged! In some cases, a prescription from a licensed physician may result in insurance reimbursement. Listed below are various protective devices that are commercially available for use in sports and/or physical activity.

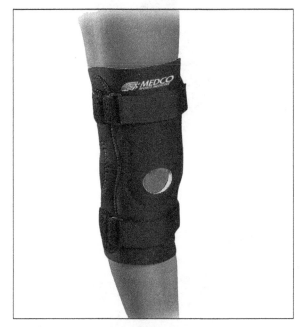

Medco Hinge Knee Brace

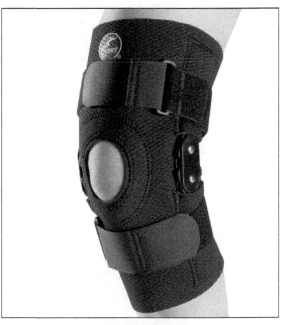

Cramer Diamond Ultralight Knee Brace

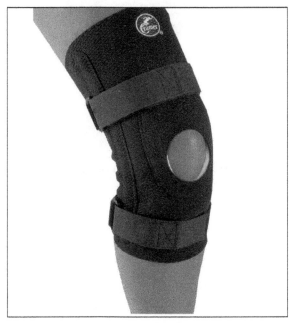

Cramer Diamond Knee Stabilizer

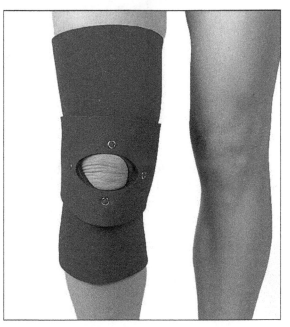

Rolyan Lateral Patella Subluxation Brace

4

4

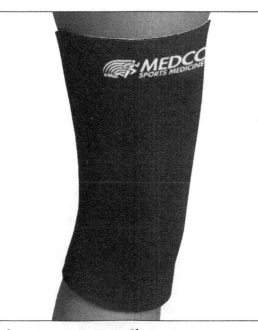

Medco Neoprene Knee Sleeve

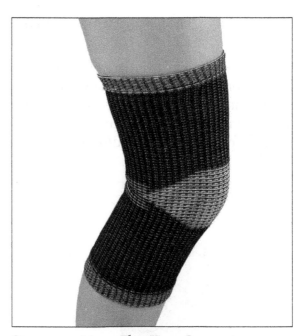

Stromgren Nano Flex Knee Support

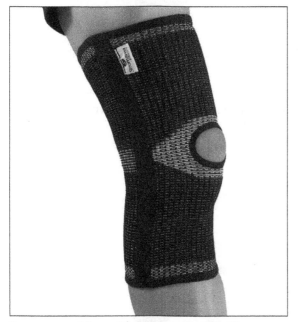

Stromgren Nano Flex Open Patella Knee
Support With Spiral Stays

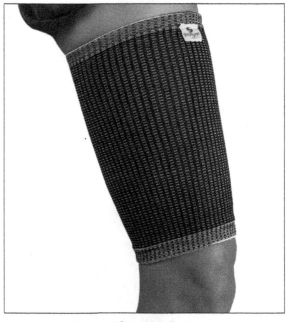

Stromgren Nano Flex Thigh Support

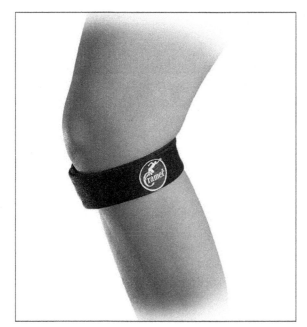

Cramer Patellar Tendon Strap

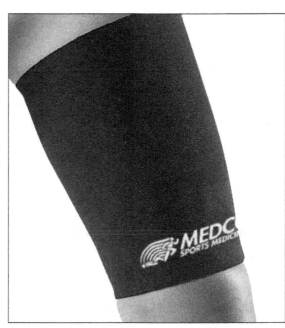

Medco Neoprene Thigh Sleeve

4

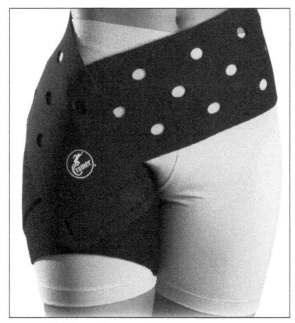

Cramer Neoprene Groin Hip Spica

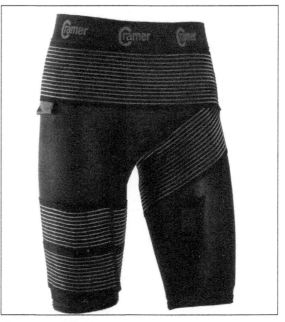

GH2 Support System

Listed below are various protective devices available to use in sport. Because a variety of protective devices is available, a qualified physician or qualified health care professional and medical equipment specialist can determine whether the individual is best suited for an off-the-shelf or custom brace.

- Osgood Schlatter condition brace
- Patella tendon strap
- Sports compression girdle

Musculoskeletal Disorders

The following is a list of common musculoskeletal disorders of the knee, thigh, and hip. For definitions of these terms, the authors encourage the learner to consult these medical references: *Taber's Medical Dictionary*, *Stedman's Medical Dictionary for the Health Professions and Nursing*, and/or *Signs and Symptoms of Athletic Injuries* (listed in Appendix B).

Knee
Anterior cruciate ligament sprain
Bursitis
Lateral collateral ligament sprain
Medial collateral ligament sprain
Meniscal tear
Myositis ossificans
Popliteal cyst
Posterior cruciate ligament sprain
Tendinitis

Thigh and Hip
Bursitis
Hip pointer
Iliotibial ossificans
Quadriceps contusion
Sprain
Strain
Tendinitis

4

Part III

The Kinesio Taping® Method

www.KinesioTaping.com

Kinesio Taping® Method

Educational Objectives

Upon completing this chapter, the reader will be able to do the following:
- Explain the purpose for selecting and using the Kinesio Taping Method
- Identify contraindications and precautions for the Kinesio Taping Method
- Demonstrate the purposes and taping procedures for the following body areas: FanCut™, foot, knee, back, neck, shoulder, and wrist

Introduction

The Kinesio Taping Method is a definitive rehabilitative taping technique that is designed to facilitate the body's natural healing process while providing support and stability to muscles and joints without restricting the body's range of motion, as well as providing extended soft tissue manipulation to prolong the benefits of manual therapy administered within the clinical setting. Latex-free and wearable for days at a time, Kinesio® Tex Tape is safe for populations ranging from pediatric to geriatric and successfully treats a variety of orthopedic, neuromuscular, neurological, and other medical conditions. The Kinesio Taping Method is a therapeutic taping technique that not only offers patients support but also rehabilitates the affected condition. By targeting different receptors within the somatosensory system, Kinesio Tex Tape alleviates pain and facilitates lymphatic drainage by microscopically lifting the skin. This lifting effect forms convolutions in the skin, thus increasing interstitial space and decreasing inflammation of the affected areas. Based upon years of clinical use, Kinesio Tex Tape is specifically applied to the patient based upon their needs after evaluation. The findings of the clinical evaluation or assessment dictate the specifics of the Kinesio Taping application and other possible treatments or modalities. With the use of single I Strips or modifications in the shape of an X, Y, or other specialized shape, and with the direction and amount of stretch placed on the tape at the time of application, Kinesio Tex Tape can be applied in hundreds of ways and has the ability to reeducate the neuromuscular system, reduce pain and inflammation, enhance performance, prevent injury and promote good circulation and healing, and assist in returning the body to homeostasis.

The Kinesio® Benefit

Evaluation and assessment are key in the treatment of any clinical condition. To achieve the desired results from a Kinesio Taping application, as well as from any other treatment, a full assessment of your patient is necessary. In some cases, the treatment of a condition may require treatment of other underlying conditions as well. This assessment should include manual muscle testing, range of motion testing, gait assessment, and any other orthopedic special tests that you deem necessary within your scope of practice. The information gained from these assessments will allow for the proper treatment protocol to be laid out. The Kinesio Taping can be a valuable addition to this protocol. It has been proven to have positive physiological effects on the skin, lymphatic, and circulatory systems, fascia, muscles, ligaments, tendons, and joints. It can be used in conjunction with a multitude of other treatments and modalities within your clinic, is effective during the rehabilitative and chronic phases of an injury, and can be used for preventative measures.

Education

Education is a key element of the Kinesio Taping Method and its continued success in the world of therapeutic taping. Along with Certified Kinesio Taping Practitioners® (CKTPs®) and Certified Kinesio Taping Instructors (CKTIs) around the world, Dr. Kase is dedicated to advancing the art and science of the method through education, clinical practice, and research. It is vital that a consistent standard of practice is maintained, and allied health professionals wishing to learn more about the Kinesio Taping Method are encouraged to participate in seminars and courses. After completing the certification program, practitioners join a select group of medical professionals who are able to properly use the Kinesio Taping Method within their realm of practice.

For more in-depth information on Kinesio Taping, contact the Kinesio Taping Association International (KTAI):

3901 Georgia Street NE, Building F
Albuquerque, NM 87110
Toll Free: (855) 488-TAPE
Phone: (505) 797-7818
www.KinesioTaping.com

Kinesio Taping
- Reeducate the neuromuscular system
- Reduce pain
- Optimize performance
- Prevent injury
- Promote improved circulation and healing

Contraindications: Do not apply Kinesio Tex Tape
- Over active malignancy site
- Over active cellulitis or skin infection
- Over open wounds, fragile or healing skin
- Over deep vein thrombosis (clots)
- If patient has had a previous skin reaction to this product

Precautions (consult with a specialist before considering applying Kinesio Taping)**:**
- Diabetes
- Kidney disease
- Lymphoedema
- Respiratory conditions
- Congestive heart failure
- CAD or bruits in the carotid artery
- Pregnancy

Kinesio Taping Don'ts

- Do not blow-dry tape
- Do not attach to nape of hair, through axilla or groin
- Do not "pull" patient into position using Kinesio® Tex Tape
- Do not touch adhesive side of tape
- Do not tape over broken skin

Kinesio Pre-Cut Methods

Fan Cut Application Instructions

The Kinesio Strip is applied using a fan cut. The crisscross pattern of the technique is applied over the area of the edema and is adjusted as needed in subsequent applications. If the lymph duct nearest to the edema is nonexistent or dysfunctional, then redirect the lymphatic fluid toward a viable duct using the anastomosis present in the lymphatic system.

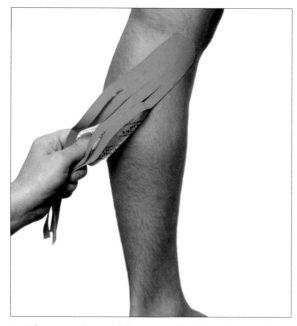

1. Place anchor of fan cut slightly above the lymph node to which lymph drainage is being directed. Have the patient move into a stretch position if appropriate for area to be treated. In example shown, the knee is in extension and the ankle in dorsiflexion.

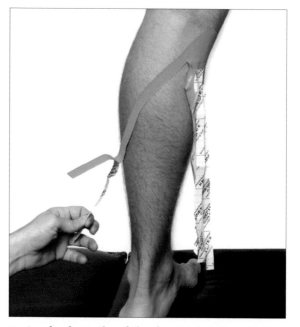

2. Apply the tails of the fan with 0% to 20% of available tension over area of edema.

5

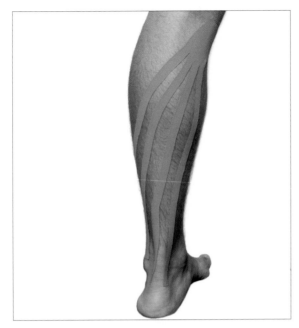

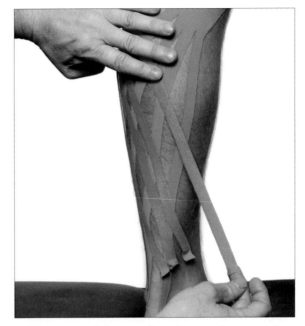

3. The placement of the lymphatic strips is directed over the area of edema. The photo shows drainage from the area of the calf to the posterior medial aspect of the knee, location of the lymph node. After the first fan cut application, pat or gently rub to activate adhesive prior to any further patient movement.

4. The second fan is placed in such a position as to create a crisscross pattern over the area of edema. Fan tails are applied using 0% to 20% of available tension.

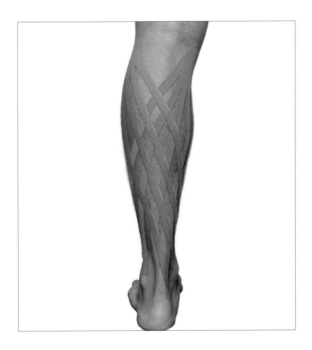

5. Following the application of the second fan strip, gently pat to initiate adhesive prior to any further patient movement. Rubbing will cause the fan strips to roll or curl, limiting wear time and effectiveness. The use of a tape adherent, bees wax, and a noncompressive tape placed on the ends may lengthen wear time.

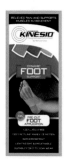

Pre-Cut Foot Instructions

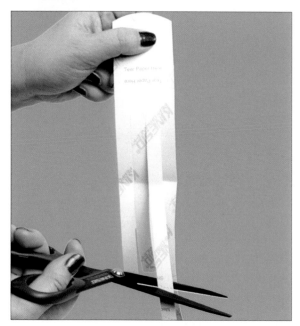 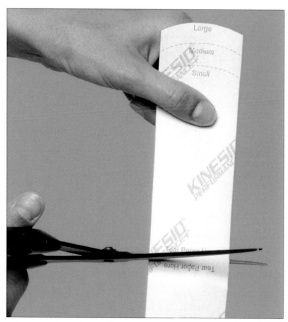

1. Take the pink tape strip and cut it to the small size using the guide on the tape backing. After cutting the strip to small, cut each tape tail in half, creating four tape tails. Take the blue tape strip and cut it in half where the tape backing indicates "tear paper here."

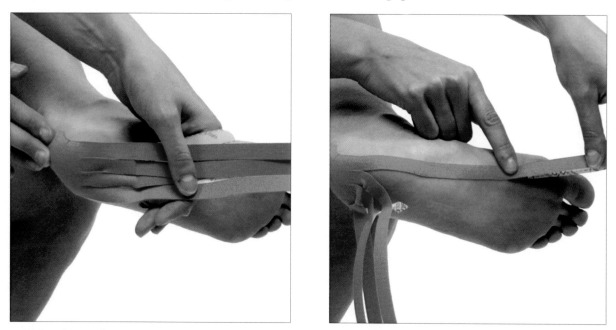

2. Take the pink tape strip and tear the paper backing where indicated on the backing paper. Remove the small section of the paper backing and apply the base of the tape strip to the back of the heel. Once applied in the correct place, the tape should be rubbed to activate the adhesive. For easier application, cut the paper backing where each tape tail begins. *Only cut the paper; do not cut the tape itself.*

5

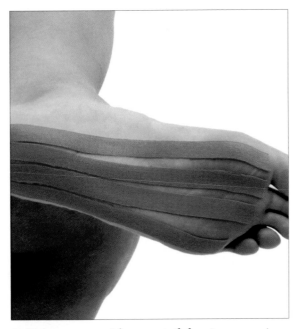

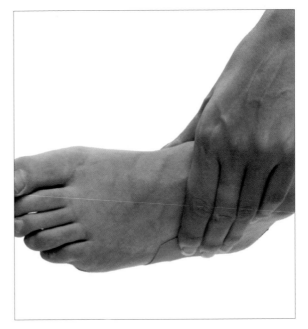

3. Using an outside tape tail, begin removing the paper backing as you apply the tape tail without stretching the tape. Repeat this process for the remaining tails so that the tape tails are spread evenly across the bottom of the foot. *Rub each tape tail to activate the adhesive.*

4. Take the blue tape strip and tear the paper backing approximately 1 in. from the end. Place the base of the blue tape strip on the outside of the foot near the center of the outside arch. Begin removing the paper backing and apply the tape strip across the bottom of the foot and pulling up on the arch with moderate tension on the tape. After the tape strip is applied to the arch, continue removing the paper backing while applying the strip to the top of the foot. The end of the tape strip should be applied without stretch. *Rub the tape to activate the adhesive.*

5

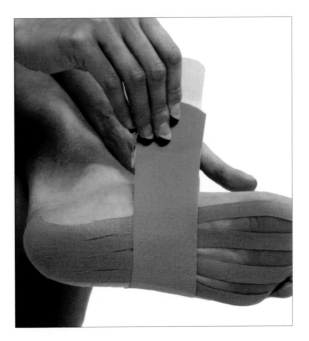

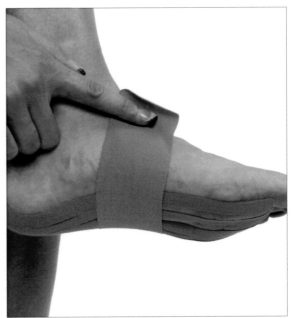

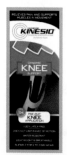

Pre-Cut Knee Instructions

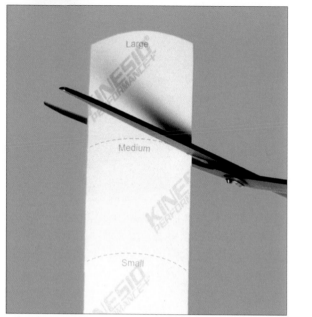

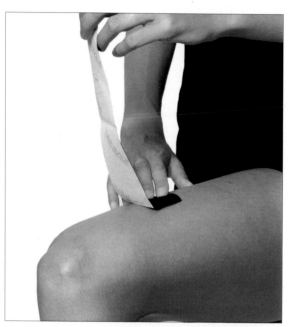

1. Take the black I strip. If required, use the guide on the tape backing to cut the strip to the correct length. Using the tear line, remove the small section of the backing paper from the base of the strip. With your knee bent to 90 degrees, place the base of the tape strip mid-thigh approximately 4 in. to 5 in. above the knee joint.

2. Without stretching the tape, begin removing the paper backing while applying the tape strip over the center of the knee joint and ending approximately 2 in. to 3 in. below the joint. *Once applied in the correct place, ub the tape to activate the adhesive.*

5

5

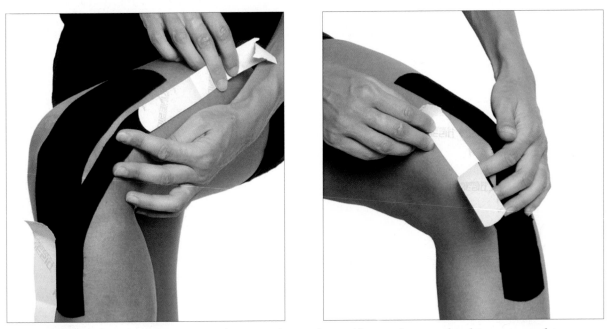

3. Take the black Y tape strip and, if required, use the guide on the tape backing to cut the tape strip to the correct length. Using the tear line, remove the paper backing and apply the base of the tape strip 2 in. to 3 in. below the knee cap. Without stretching the tape, apply each tape tail around each side of the knee joint. *Rub the tape to activate the adhesive.*

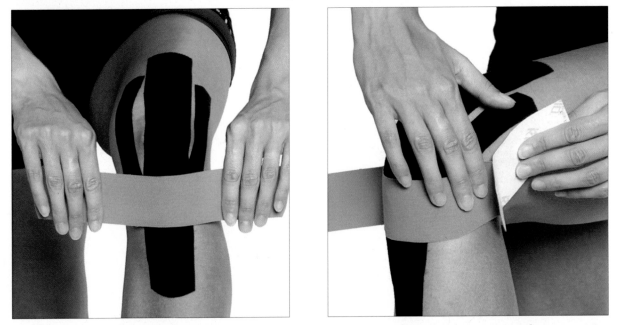

4. Take the blue tape strip and, if required, use the guide on the tape backing to cut the tape strip to the correct length. Using the tear line, remove the paper backing halfway down each side of the tape strip to expose the middle of the adhesive. Using minimal stretch, apply the middle portion just below the knee cap. Apply the remaining sides without stretch. *Rub the tape to activate the adhesive.*

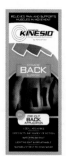

Pre-Cut Back Instructions

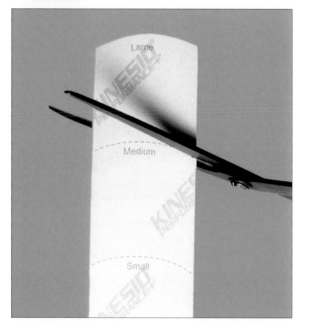

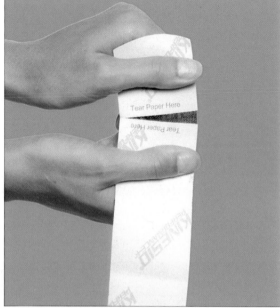

5

1. Take one black tape strip and, if required, use the guide on the tape backing to cut the strip to the correct length. Using the tear line, remove the small section of the backing paper from the strip.

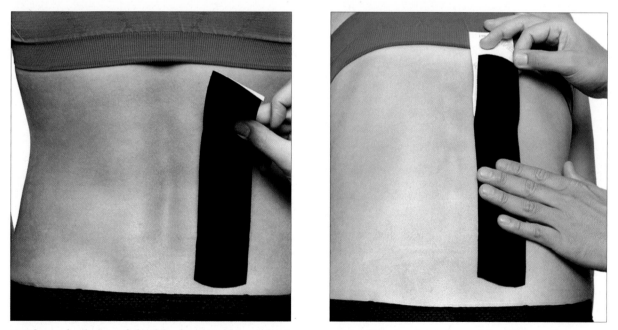

2. Place the base of the black strip above the lowest part of the back on one side of the spine. Bend forward to stretch the back muscles and begin removing tape backing. Without stretching the tape, extend the strip up and alongside the spine. *Once applied in the correct place, rub the tape to activate the adhesive.*

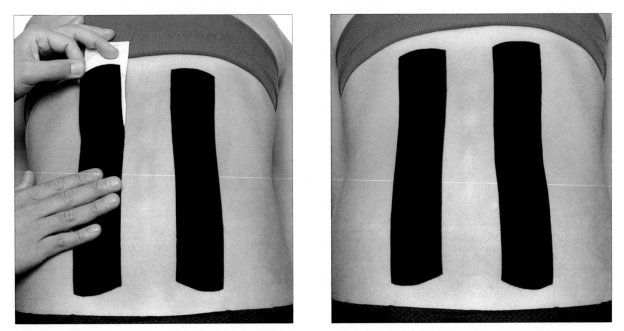

3. Take the other black strip and repeat the previous step for the opposite side of the spine. *Rub the tape to activate the adhesive.*

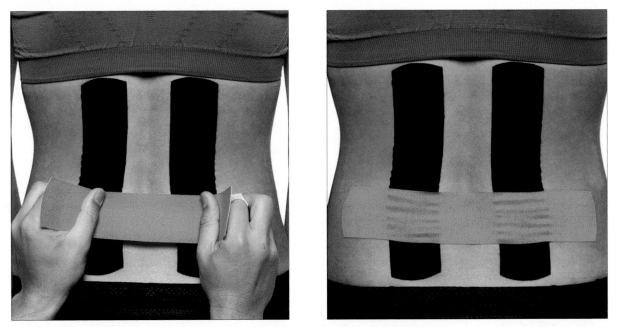

4. Take the pink strip and, if required, use the guide on the tape backing to cut the tape strip to the correct length. Using the tear line, remove the paper backing halfway down each side of the strip to expose the middle portion of the adhesive. Using minimal tension, apply the tape strip horizontally over the strained area on the lower back. *Rub the tape to activate the adhesive.*

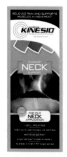

Pre-Cut Neck Instructions

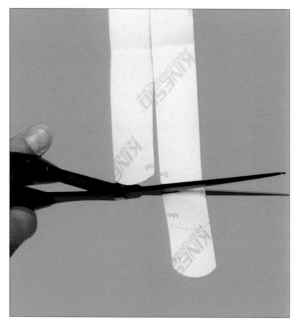

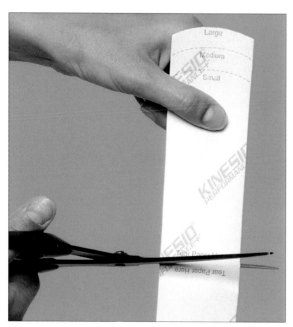

5

1. Take the beige tape strip and cut it to the small size using the guide on the tape backing. Take the black tape strip and cut it in half where the tape backing indicates "tear paper here."

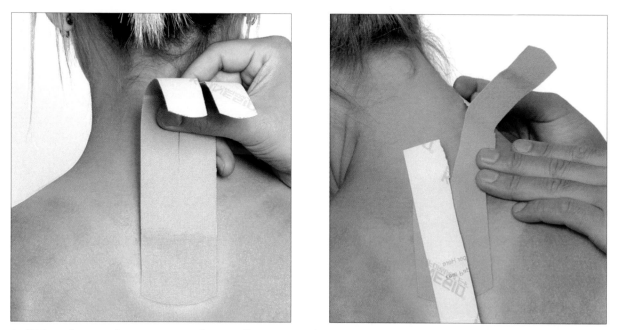

2. Using the tear line, remove the small section of the tape backing. Place the base of the tape strip in the center of the spine about 2 in. to 3 in. below the base of the neck. Tilt your head forward and to the left. Begin applying the right tape tail up the right side of the neck. Be careful not to apply the tape tail over loose hair. *Once applied in the correct place, rub the tape to activate the adhesive.*

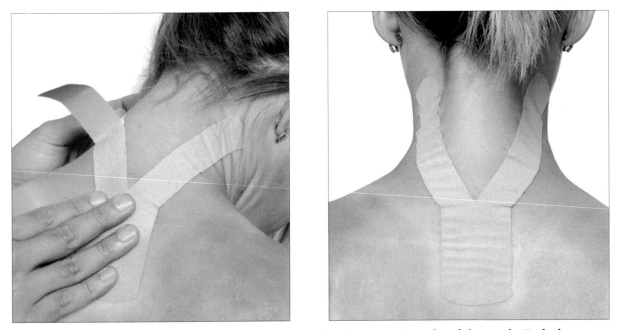

3. Using the left tape tail, repeat the previous step for the opposite side of the neck. *Rub the tape to activate the adhesive.*

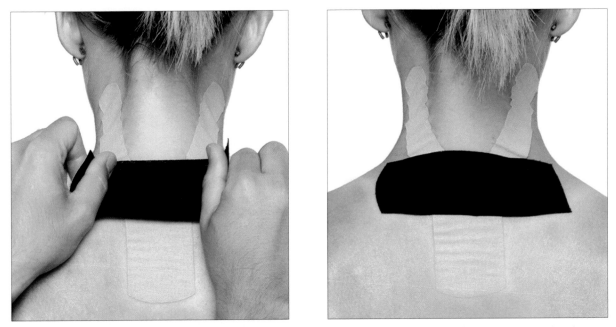

4. Take one of the black tape strips and fold it in half. After folding in half, tear the tape backing in the center of the tape strip. Remove the tape backing halfway down each side of the tape strip to expose the center portion of the adhesive. Using minimal tension, apply the tape strip over the strained portion of the neck. Apply ends without stretch. *Rub the tape to activate the adhesive.*

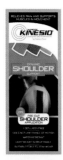

Pre-Cut Shoulder Instructions

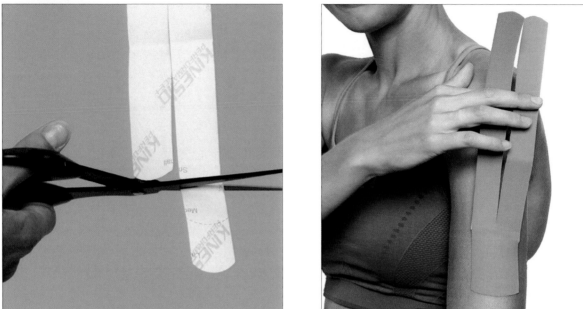

5

1. Take one blue Y tape strip and, if required, use the guide on the tape backing to cut the strip to the correct length. Using the tear line, remove the small section of the paper backing from the tape strip and apply the base of the tape strip at the midpoint of the arm.

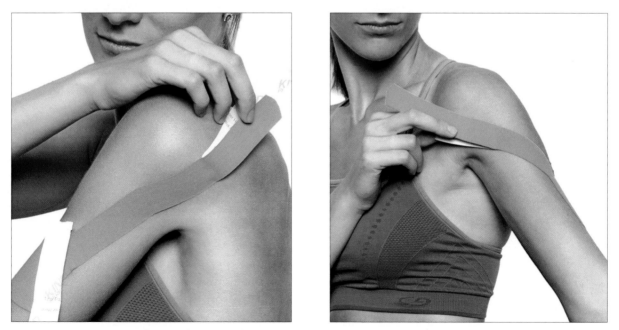

2. Move your arm in front of you, and without stretching the tape, apply the back tape tail along the back of your shoulder. Once applied in the correct place, both tape tails should be rubbed to activate the adhesive. Move your arm back at a 45-degree angle, and without stretching the tape, apply the front tape tail along the front of your shoulder. *Rub the tape to activate the adhesive.*

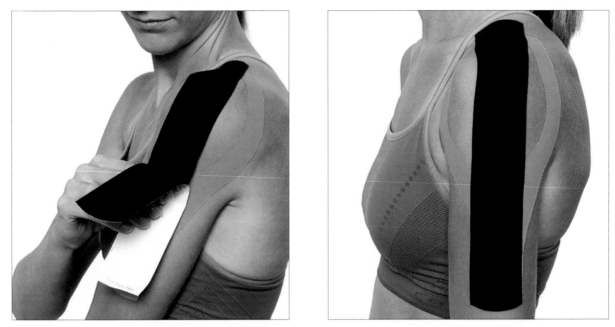

3. Take the black tape strip and, if required, use the guide on the tape backing to cut the tape strip to the correct length. Using the tear line, remove the paper backing and apply the base of the tape strip approximately 3 in. to 4 in. above the shoulder joint. Without stretching the tape, apply the tape strip over the shoulder joint and down the arm, ending over the base of the blue Y tape strip. *Rub the tape to activate the adhesive.*

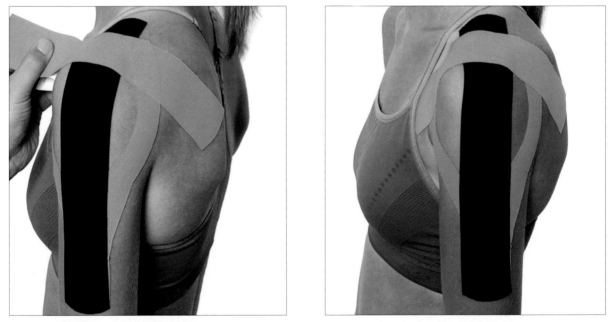

4. OPTIONAL (for more support): Take the remaining blue tape strip and, if required, use the guide on the tape backing to cut the tape strip to the correct length. With assistance, using the tear line, remove the paper backing and apply the base to the shoulder blade. Begin removing the remaining paper backing and apply the tape strip over the shoulder joint without stretching the tape. *Rub the tape to activate the adhesive.*

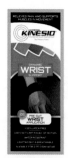

Pre-Cut Wrist Instructions

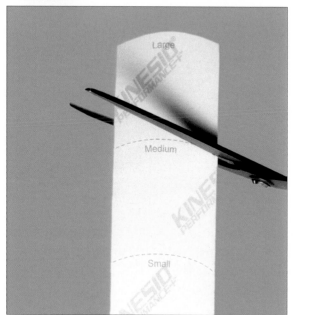

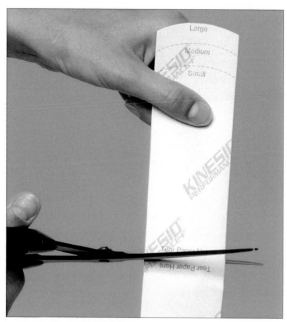

5

1. Take one blue tape strip and, if required, use the guide on the tape backing to cut the strip to the correct length. Take the black tape strip and cut it in half where the tape backing indicates "tear paper here."

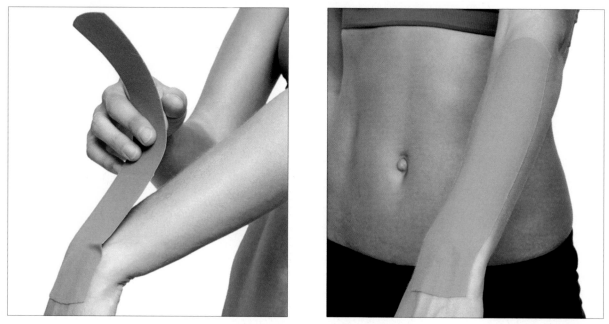

2. Using the blue tape strip, tear the paper backing where indicated on the tape backing. Remove the small section of the tape backing. Bend the wrist/hand downward and place the base of the blue tape strip above the knuckles. Without stretching the tape, begin removing the remaining paper backing as you apply the tape strip over the wrist joint and up the arm. *Once applied in the correct place, rub the tape to activate the adhesive.*

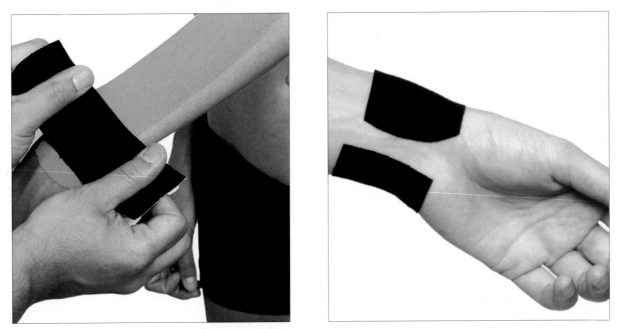

3. Take one black tape strip and fold it in half. After folding it in half, tear the tape backing in the center of the tape strip. Remove the tape backing halfway down each side of the tape strip to expose the middle portion of the adhesive. With assistance, apply the tape strip over the top of the wrist joint using minimal stretch. Apply ends with no stretch around wrist joint so that they do not overlap. *Rub the tape to activate the adhesive.*

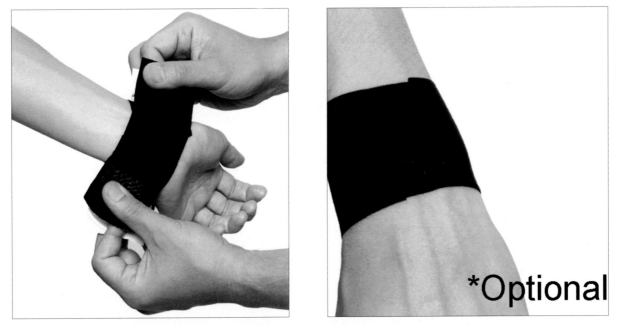

*Optional

4. OPTION 1 (for more support): Using a second black tape strip, repeat the previous step but apply the tape strip to the bottom of the wrist joint. *Rub the tape to activate the adhesive.* OPTION 2: Using two black tape strips, repeat Step 3 and Option 1. Option 2 is only used to achieve support for the wrist joint if applied without the blue I tape. *Rub the tape to activate the adhesive.*

Part IV

Techniques for
Upper Extremities

6 Shoulder and Upper Arm

Educational Objectives

Upon completing this chapter, the reader will be able to do the following:
- Identify anatomical landmarks critical for correct taping procedures
- Describe the purpose for the applications of adhesive and elastic tape
- Select the proper supplies and specialty items used for taping
- Explain the steps in preparing the body for taping, wrapping, or protective device
- Describe and demonstrate the purposes, clinical applications, anatomical structures, supplies needed, and pre-taping and taping procedures for anatomical areas
- Identify the proper use and application of protective devices for the shoulder and upper arm

Introduction

The shoulder and upper arm can be complex to understand due the multiple movements. The occurrence of an injury to the area can compound the complexity. In this chapter, terminology, taping techniques, wrapping techniques, protective devices, and musculoskeletal disorders to the shoulder and upper arm will be discussed to provide greater clarity.

Terminology

External rotation. Turning outwardly or away from the midline of the body.

Internal rotation. Turning inwardly or toward the midline of the body.

Abduction. Lateral movement of a limb away from the median plane of the body; movement away from the median plane around an anterior–posterior axis with the angle between the displaced parts becoming greater, as in lifting the arm sideward away from the body.

Adduction. Lateral movement of a limb toward the median plane of the body; movement toward the median plane around an anterior–posterior axis with the angle between the displaced parts becoming lesser, as in bringing the arm sideward against the body.

Circumduction. Movement around an axis such that the proximal end of a limb is fixed and the distal end traces a circle.

Shoulder and Upper Arm

Taping and Wrapping Techniques and Protective Devices

Developing a thorough knowledge regarding the fundamentals about the application of taping/wrapping procedures is imperative. Review Chapter 1 before applying any technique.

Proper Assessment of Injury

Before applying a preventive technique (tape, wrap, and/or device), a qualified physician must complete a proper injury evaluation. Following the injury evaluation, a qualified health care professional can then recommend proper taping techniques. This ensures that proper taping techniques are applied for support and stabilization. Also, developing a thorough knowledge of taping application fundamentals is imperative.

Purpose and Application of Adhesive and Elastic Tape

The primary purpose for tape application is to provide additional support and stability for the affected body part. Through proper application, taping techniques can be applied to shorten the muscle's angle of pull; to decrease joint range of motion; to secure pads, bandages, and protective devices; and to apply compression to reduce swelling.

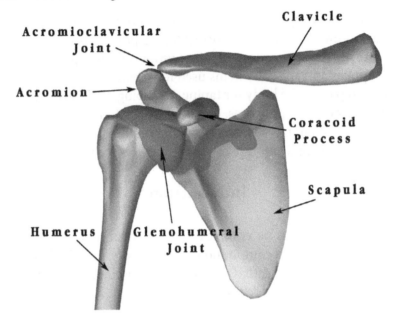

Figure 6.1. Bony anatomy of the upper arm and shoulder

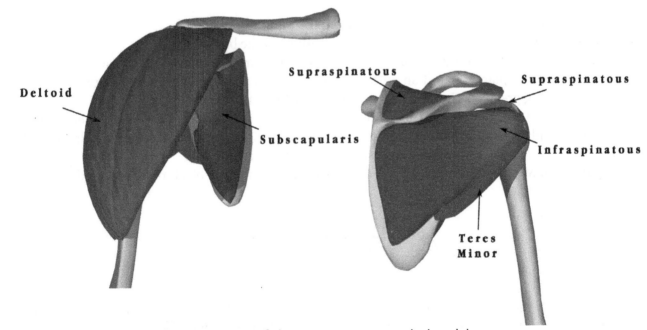

Figure 6.2. Muscular anatomy of the upper arm and shoulder

Medical Supplies and Specialty Items

Purchasing supplies depends on budget, philosophy of medical staff regarding taping techniques, and occurrence of injury. Review Chapter 1 before applying any technique.

Specific Rules on Taping, Wrapping, and/or Protective Device

If you apply supportive techniques to an individual, you should be aware of specific rules governing tape application in that particular sport or physical activity. Your application must fall within the guidelines established for each sport by appropriate governing bodies.

Special Techniques: Adjunct Taping Procedures

The taping techniques presented are the fundamental procedures. Adjunct techniques will be shown to provide additional support; however, you should still follow the fundamental procedures. Variations can be achieved by adapting these techniques to a particular injury situation. Always give special consideration to

- purpose of the taping procedure
- clinical application
- correct anatomical position
- supply selection
- tape/wrap technique or protective device

Preparation of Body Part for Taping

In preparing the body for tape application, consider these items:

1. removal of hair (optional)
2. clean the area
3. special considerations
4. spray adherent (optional)
5. skin lubricants
6. underwrap or cohesive tape

Proper Body Position

Before beginning a taping procedure, select a comfortable table height and ask the individual to assume an anatomically correct and comfortable position.

6

- Neutral Position of Shoulder—Acromioclavicular Joint: The individual should be in a standing position with shoulder abducted, elbow flexed, hand set on waist, and chest slightly expanded.
- Neutral Position of Shoulder—Glenohumeral Joint: The individual should stand with should abducted, elbow flexed, and bicep muscles contracts, hand set on low back and chest expanded.

When applying a technique, learn to stand at a comfortable and stationary position and place the body part to be taped at your elbow height.

Taping Techniques

The taping techniques presented are the fundamental procedures. A strong knowledge of anatomy, physiology, and biomechanics is essential. Developing a thorough knowledge regarding the fundamentals about the application of taping/wrapping procedures is imperative. Review Section A - Chapter 1 before applying any technique.

Acromioclavicular (AC) Joint

Purpose:	To provide support and stabilization to the acromioclavicular (AC) joint
Clinical Application:	Sprains and contusions
Anatomical Structure:	Acromioclavicular joint of the shoulder
Anatomical Position:	The individual should be in a standing position with shoulder abducted, elbow flexed, hand set on waist, and chest slightly expanded.
Supplies:	2-in. elastic tape, 1½-in. adhesive tape, and gauze pad or large Band-Aid

6

Pre-Taping Procedure:

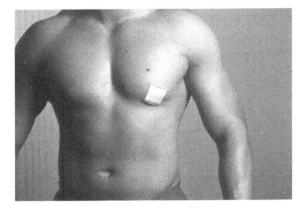

Place the gauze pad or Band-Aid over the nipple of the affected side.

Taping Procedures:

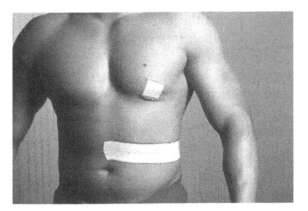

1. Using 2-in. elastic tape, place a horizontal anchor strip from the anterior to the posterior body midline. This anchor strip should cover the mid- or lower portion of the rib cage.

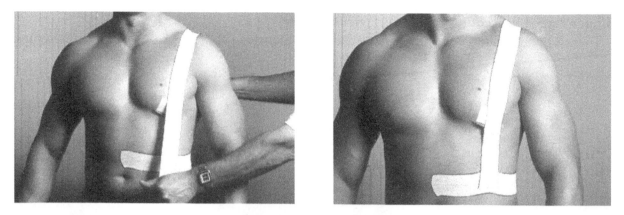

2. Measure the distance from the anterior portion of the anchor across the AC joint and end on the posterior anchor. Apply a strip of 1½-in. adhesive tape to this area. With the middle of the tape placed on the AC joint, apply equal tension toward both the anterior end and the posterior end and attach tape to the anchor.

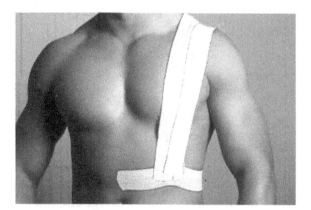

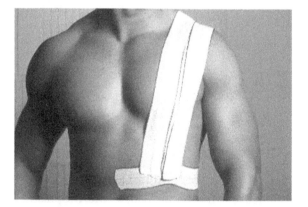

3. Repeat step 2 three times.

6

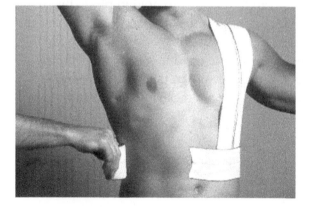

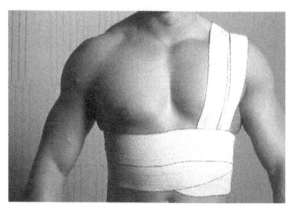

4. To add additional support, encircle a second horizontal anchor strip around the torso.

*Upon completion of the procedure, make sure you check for neatness and gaps, adequate support, along with proper function of the affected area. In certain situations, the individual might be asked to perform function tests to establish appropriate technique application.

Adjunct Taping Procedures: Acromioclavicular Joint

These adjunct taping procedures can be used in conjunction with the basic technique presented.

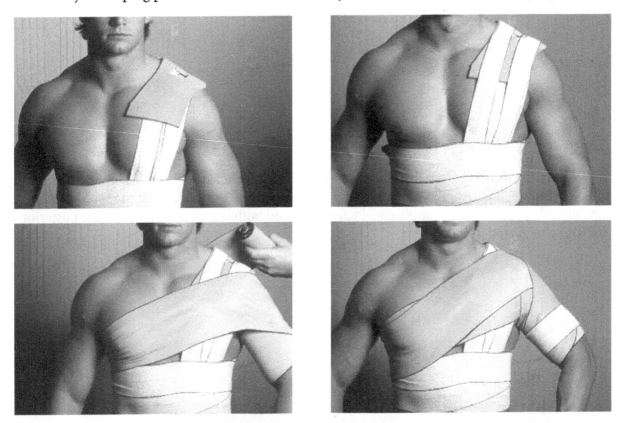

Technique A. For additional protection to the AC joint, construct a felt or foam rubber pad that is at least ½ in. thick. Also, a "thermoplastic" pad may be used! The pad must be large enough to cover the affected superior aspect of the shoulder. Cut a hole in this protective pad and place over the affected AC joint. To secure this pad, apply 2-in. elastic tape over the AC joint. Using a 6-in. extra long elastic wrap, apply a shoulder spica wrap to this area to hold in place. Begin on the posterior aspect of the upper arm, move anteriorly, encircle the arm, continue across the anterior aspect of the chest, go under the opposite arm, go across the posterior aspect of the torso angling upward and over the affected AC joint, and encircle the upper arm. Repeat this procedure a second time. Secure the wrap with 2-in. elastic tape. When taping the FEMALE INDIVIDUAL, apply this procedure the same; however, the horizontal strips should end above the breast.

6

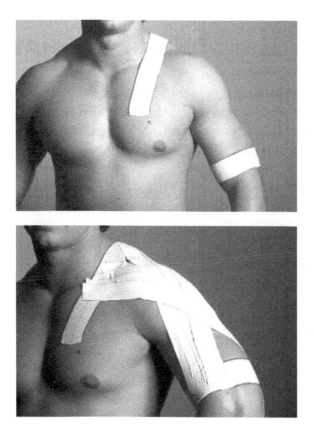

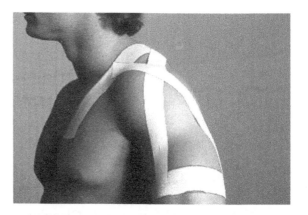

Technique B. For individuals who have difficulty in the complete application of this technique around the shoulder girdle and torso, a modified version can be applied. After placing the horizontal anchor strip in the mid-region of the chest, apply stability strips with equal tension toward the anterior and posterior anchors strips. Repeat this step four times, and then anchor for stability.

6

Glenohumeral Joint

Purpose:	To provide support and stability to the glenohumeral joint of the shoulder. A continuous strip of elastic tape is applied in a shoulder spica method. This supportive technique should restrict abduction and external rotation of the glenohumeral joint.
Clinical Application:	Sprains and strains
Anatomical Structure:	Glenohumeral joint
Anatomical Position:	The individual should stand with shoulder abducted, elbow flexed, biceps muscles contracted, hand set on low back, and chest expanded
Supplies:	3-in. elastic tape and gauze pads or Band-Aid

Pre-Taping Procedure:

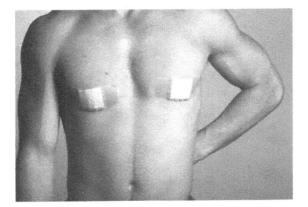

Cover both nipples with gauze pads or Band-Aid

Taping Procedures:

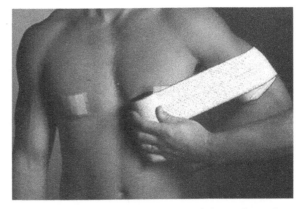

1. Begin on the distal aspect of the affected upper arm, move anteriorly, encircle the arm, continue across the anterior aspect of the chest, go under the opposite arm, go across the posterior aspect of the torso, and encircle the distal aspect of the upper arm.

6

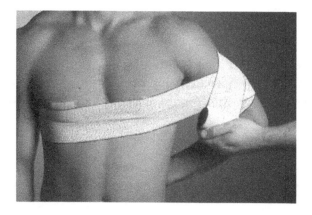

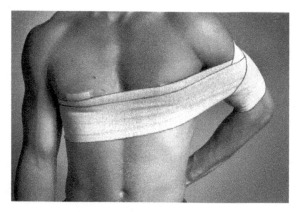

2. Repeat this procedure a second time.
Comment: In certain situations, a check rein can be applied between the torso and upper arm. This technique will aid in preventing the glenohumeral joint from excessive abduction and external rotation.

*Upon completion of the procedure, make sure you check for neatness and gaps, adequate support, along with proper function of the affected area. In certain situations, the individual might be asked to perform function tests to establish appropriate technique application.

Adjunct Taping Procedure: Glenohumeral Joint
These adjunct taping procedures can be used in conjunction with the basic technique presented.

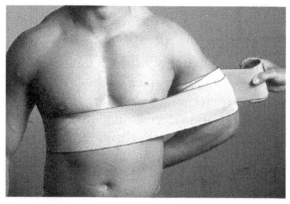

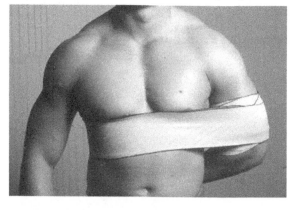

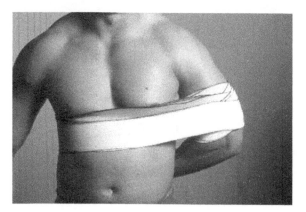

Technique A. Using a 6-in. extra long elastic wrap, apply a shoulder spica wrap to this area. This support wrap should restrict abduction and external rotation of the shoulder. Begin on the posterior aspect of the upper arm, move anteriorly, encircle the arm, continue across the anterior aspect of the chest, go under the opposite arm, go across the posterior aspect of the torso angling upward, go over the affected joint, and then encircle the upper arm. Repeat this procedure a second time. Secure the wrap by using a continuous strip of elastic tape in the same pattern as the wrap.

6

Wrapping Techniques for Support

During physical activity, supportive wraps are used to aid in muscle function and support and to reduce excessive range of motion. These applications are typically used in competition or practice. Spica wraps are traditionally employed at the hip and shoulder joints. Figure of 8 wraps are placed over ankle, knee, elbow, wrist, and hand joints.

Glenohumeral Joint Wrap

Purpose:	To provide support to the glenohumeral joint of the shoulder
Clinical Application:	Sprains of the glenohumeral joint
Anatomical Structure:	Glenohumeral joint
Anatomical Position:	The individual should stand with shoulder abducted, elbow flexed, biceps muscle contracted, and hand set on hip or low back.
Supplies:	6-in. extra long elastic wrap and 2-in. adhesive tape
Pre-Wrapping Procedure:	The individual should breathe deeply, expanding the chest. Then you can begin the wrap.

Wrapping Procedures:

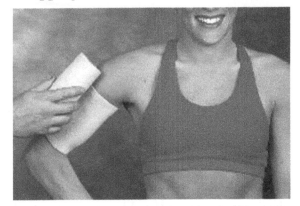

1. Apply a continuous strip of 6-in. elastic wrap in a shoulder spica method. This supportive technique should restrict abduction and external rotation of the glenohumeral joint. Begin on the distal aspect of the biceps muscle of the affected arm, move anteriorly, and encircle the arm.

6

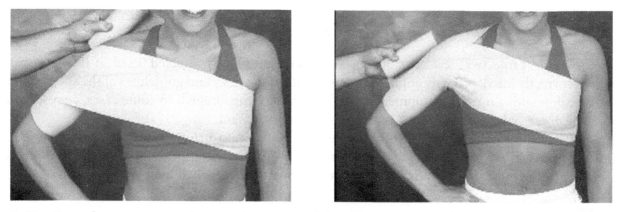

2. Continue the wrap across the anterior aspect of the chest, go under the opposite arm, go across the posterior aspect of the torso, and encircle the distal aspect of the upper arm.

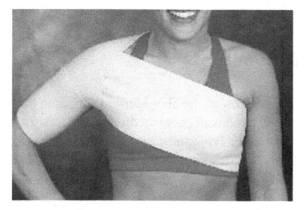

3. Repeat this procedure a second time.

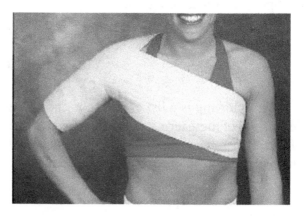

4. Secure the wrap by using a continuous strip of elastic tape in the same pattern as the wrap. Anchor the wrap with 2-in. elastic tape following the same pattern as the wrap.

*Upon completion of the procedure, make sure you check for neatness and gaps, adequate support, along with proper function of the affected area. In certain situations, the individual might be asked to perform function tests to establish appropriate technique application.

6

Protective Devices

The use of protective devices is beneficial if they are properly selected, used in the appropriate setting, correctly fitted, properly applied, and used within the rules and guidelines of the specific sport. Consultation with a medical equipment specialist is highly encouraged! In some cases, a prescription from a licensed physician may result in insurance reimbursement.

Listed below are various protective devices available to use in sport. Because a variety of protective devices are availabe, a qualified physician or qualified health care professional and medical equipment specialist can determine whether the individual is best suited for an off-the-shelf or custom brace

- AC Joint Pad
- Blockers exostosis pad
- Glenohumeral joint stailizer brace
- Sports compression girdle
- Sternum protector

Musculoskeletal Disorders

The following is a list of common musculoskeletal disorders of the shoulder and upper arm. For definitions of these terms, the authors encourage the learner to consult these medical references: *Taber's Medical Dictionary*, *Stedman's Medical Dictionary for the Health Professions and Nursing*, and/or *Signs and Symptoms of Athletic Injuries* (listed in Appendix B).

Shoulder and Upper Arm

Blockers exostosis	Separation
Bursitis	Sprain
Contusion	Strain
Dislocation	Subluxation
Nerve injury	Synovitis
Rotator cuff dysfunction	Tendonitis
Rotator cuff impingement	Tenosynovitis
Rotator cuff strain	

6

Elbow, Forearm, Wrist, and Hand

Educational Objectives

Upon completing this chapter, the reader will be able to do the following:
- Identify anatomical landmarks critical for correct taping procedures
- Describe the purpose for the applications of adhesive and elastic tape
- Select the proper supplies and specialty items used for taping
- Explain the steps in preparing the body for taping, wrapping, or protective device
- Describe and demonstrate the purposes, clinical applications, anatomical structures, supplies needed, and pre-taping and taping procedures for anatomical areas
- Identify the proper use and application of protective devices for the elbow, forearm, wrist, and hand

Introduction

The ability to use the elbow, forearm, wrist, and hand for active use is important for daily living. Nevertheless, the occurrence of an injury is possible and can be problematic. This chapter will cover terminology, taping techniques, wrapping techniques, protective devices, and musculoskeletal disorders for the elbow, forearm, wrist, and hand to assist with injury care.

Terminology

Flexion. Movement around a transverse axis in an anterior–posterior plane with the angle between the anterior aspects of the displaced parts becoming smaller, as in bending the forearm toward the arm at the elbow joint; the act of drawing a body segment away from a straight line with its proximally conjoined body segment or toward that smallest acute angle of the joint.

Extension. The reverse movement during which the angle between the anterior aspects of the displaced parts is increased, as in moving the forearm away from the upper arm; the act of drawing a body segment toward a straight line position with its proximally conjoined body segment or away from the body joint.

Pronation. Act of rotating the hand or foot internally on its long axis; medial rotation of the forearm, as in turning the palm of the hand downward.

Supination. Act of rotating the hand or foot externally on its long axis; lateral rotation of the forearm, as in turning the palm of the hand upward

Anatomical snuffbox. Space at the base of the thumb created by the extensor pollicis longus and brevis tendons.

Elbow, Forearm, Wrist, and Hand

Taping and Wrapping Techniques and Protective Devices

Developing a thorough knowledge regarding the fundamentals about the application of taping/wrapping procedures is imperative. Review Chapter 1 before applying any technique.

Proper Assessment of Injury

Before applying a preventive technique (tape, wrap, and/or device), a qualified physician should complete a proper injury evaluation. Following the injury evaluation, a qualified health care professional can then recommend proper taping techniques. This ensures that proper taping techniques are applied for support and stabilization. Also, developing a thorough knowledge of taping application fundamentals is imperative.

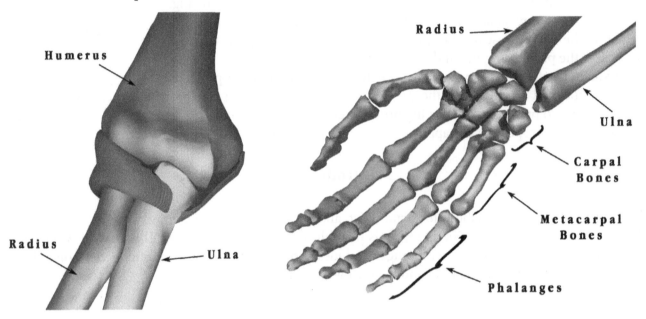

Figure 7.1. Bony anatomy of the elbow, forearm, wrist, and hand.

7

Purpose and Application of Adhesive and Elastic Tape

The primary purpose for tape application is to provide additional support and stability for the affected body part. Through proper application, taping techniques can be applied to shorten the muscle's angle of pull; to decrease joint range of motion; to secure pads, bandages, and protective devices; and to apply compression to reduce swelling.

Medical Supplies and Specialty Items

Purchasing supplies depends on budget, philosophy of medical staff regarding taping techniques, and occurrence of injury. Review Chapter 1 before applying any technique.

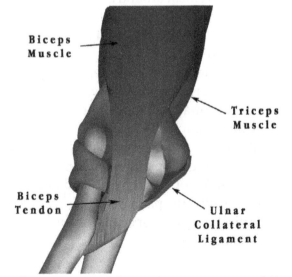

Figure 7.2. Muscular anatomy of the elbow and forearm.

Specific Rules on Taping, Wrapping, and/or Protective Device

If you apply supportive techniques to an individual, you should be aware of specific rules governing tape application in that particular sport or physical activity. Your application must fall within the guidelines established for each sport by appropriate governing bodies.

Special Techniques: Adjunct Taping Procedures

The taping techniques presented are the fundamental procedures. Adjunct techniques will be shown to provide additional support; however, you should still follow the fundamental procedures. Variations can be achieved by adapting these techniques to a particular injury situation. Always give special consideration to

- purpose of the taping procedure
- clinical application
- correct anatomical position
- supply selection
- tape/wrap technique or protective device

Preparation of Body Part for Taping

In preparing the body for tape application, consider these items:

1. removal of hair (optional)
2. clean the area
3. special considerations
4. spray adherent (optional)
5. skin lubricants
6. underwrap or cohesive tape

Proper Body Positioning

Before beginning a taping procedure, select a comfortable table height and ask the individual to assume an anatomically correct and comfortable position.

- Neutral Position of Elbow: From the anatomical position, the elbow joint should be held in slight flexion (10 to 15 degrees).
- Neutral Position of Wrist and Hand: This position can vary, so consult specific taping techniques for anatomical structure placement.

When applying a technique, learn to stand at a comfortable and stationary position and place the body part to be taped at your elbow height.

Taping and Wrapping Techniques

The taping techniques presented are the fundamental procedures. A strong knowledge of anatomy, physiology, and biomechanics is essential. Developing a thorough knowledge regarding the fundamentals about the application of taping/wrapping procedures is imperative. Review Section 1 - Chapter 1 before applying any technique.

7

Elbow Hyperextension

Purpose:	To provide support and stability to the elbow joint
Clinical Application:	Sprains and strains
Anatomical Structure:	Elbow
Anatomical Position:	Forearm supinated and in slight flexion
Supplies:	2-in. elastic tape and 1½-in. adhesive tape

VIDEO

Taping Procedures:

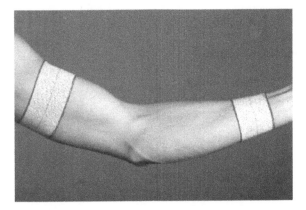

1. Apply two anchor strips of 2-in. elastic tape. Position the proximal anchor above the belly of the biceps muscle and the distal anchor on the distal one third of the forearm.

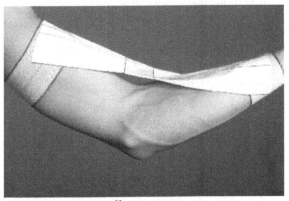

2. Using 1½-in. adhesive tape, construct a five- to seven-strip butterfly. Prior to application, place a strip of tape around the mid-portion of this support pattern. Apply the butterfly pattern from the proximal anchor to the distal anchor. Apply proper tension to ensure that the elbow does not reach full extension.

7

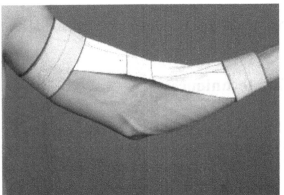

3. Apply a second series of anchor strips using elastic tape.

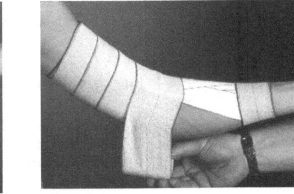

4. Apply a final continuous closure strip with 2-in. elastic tape. Beginning on the distal anchor, spiral the tape, overlapping one half of its width, and end on the proximal anchor.

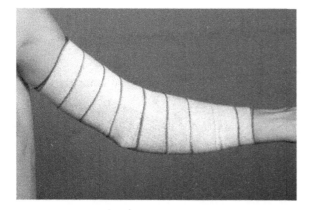

*Upon completion of the procedure, make sure you check for neatness and gaps, adequate support, along with proper function of the affected area. In certain situations, the individual might be asked to perform function tests to establish appropriate technique application.

Adjunct Taping Procedure: Elbow Hyperextension

These adjunct taping procedures can be used in conjunction with the basic technique presented.

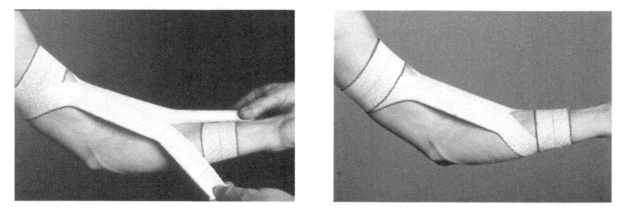

Technique A. This technique aids in preventing the elbow joint from excessive extension. Using 2-in. elastic tape, cut a strip 9 in. to 12 in. in length, split both ends lengthwise approximately 3 in. With the elbow in slight flexion, encircle the proximal anchor with the split ends of the elastic tape. Pull the tape to full tension and encircle the distal anchor with the other split end of the elastic tape. Apply 2-in. elastic tape to secure the anchors.

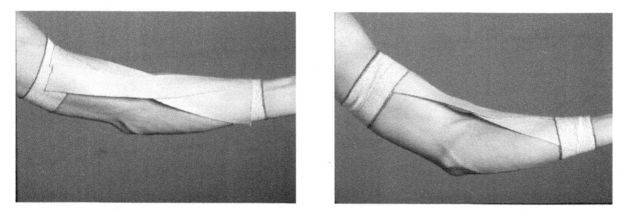

Technique B. Use adhesive felt in place of the adhesive tape butterfly pattern.

7

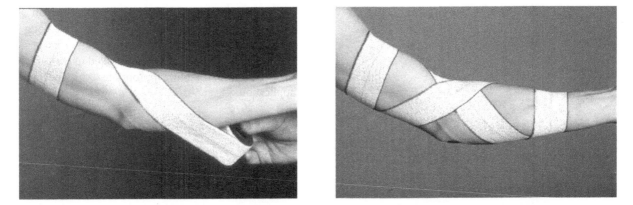

Technique C. Apply a figure of 8 pattern using 2-in. elastic tape. Beginning on the anterior lateral aspect of the upper arm, cross the elbow joint at the medial epicondyle, encircle the forearm, cross the lateral epicondyle, and anchor on the anterior medial aspect of the upper arm. Use caution to avoid circulatory dysfunction.

7

Elbow Epicondylitis

Purpose: To help reduce the pain associated with epicondylitis

Clinical Application: Epicondylitis

Anatomical Structure: Elbow

Anatomical Position:
- Medial epicondylitis: Elbow extended and forearm supinated
- Lateral epicondylitis: Elbow extended and forearm pronated

Supplies: 2-in. elastic tape, 1-in. adhesive tape, and ½-in. or ⅜-in. felt pad

Pre-Taping Procedures: Cut felt to cover affected area.

Taping Procedures:

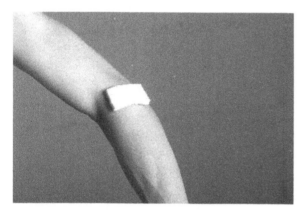

1. Place felt pad over affected area.

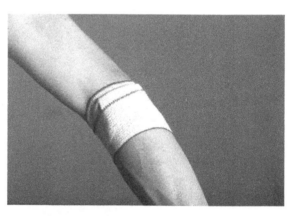

2. Anchor the felt pad using elastic tape. Encircle the forearm two or three times.

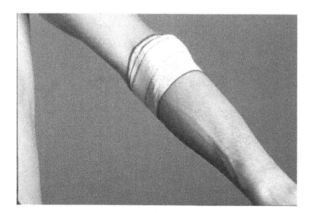

3. Secure the elastic tape ends with two or three support strips of adhesive tape, overlapping the tape by one half of its width.

*Upon completion of the procedure, make sure you check for neatness and gaps, adequate support, along with proper function of the affected area. In certain situations, the individual might be asked to perform function tests to establish appropriate technique application.

7

Adjunct Taping Procedure: Elbow Epicondylitis

These adjunct taping procedures can be used in conjunction with the basic technique presented.

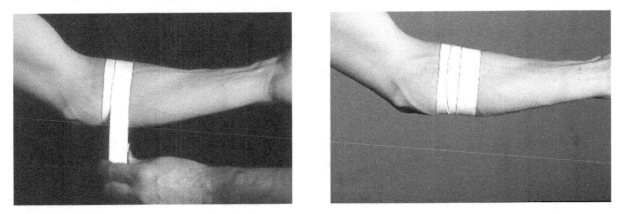

Technique A. Use 1-in. adhesive tape to apply two to three circular strips approximately 2 in. below the condyles of the elbow.

7

Forearm Splint

Purpose:	To help reduce the pain associated with forearm splints
Clinical Application:	Forearm splints
Anatomical Structure:	Forearm
Anatomical Position:	Elbow joint placed in slight flexion (10 to 15 degrees)
Supplies:	1½-in. adhesive tape and 2-in. elastic tape

Taping Procedures:

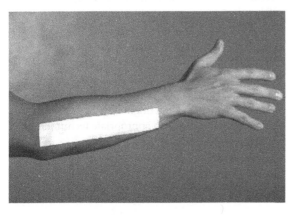

1. Apply anchor strips on the medial and lateral aspects of the forearm using 1½-in. adhesive tape.

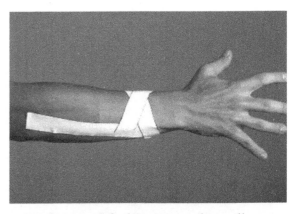

2. Apply a modified X pattern that will cover the affected area. Begin on the distal ends of the anchors and work toward the proximal ends.

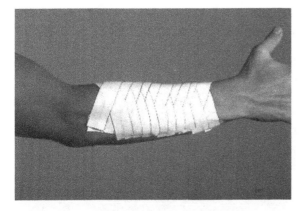

3. Apply three to six sets of X patterns, overlapping the tape by one half of its width.

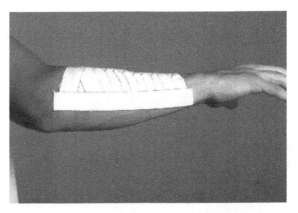

4. Apply a second set of anchors to help hold the technique in place. Do not cover the posterior aspect of the forearm with adhesive tape.

7

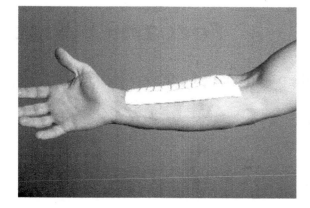

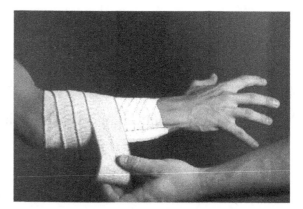

5. Apply a final continuous closure strip with 2-in. elastic tape. Begin on the proximal anchor and spiral the tape, overlapping the tape by one half of its width, and end on the distal anchor. Secure the elastic tape ends with adhesive tape anchors.

*Upon completion of the procedure, make sure you check for neatness and gaps, adequate support, along with proper function of the affected area. In certain situations, the individual might be asked to perform function tests to establish appropriate technique application.

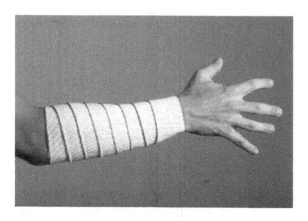

Adjunct Taping Procedure: Forearm Strain
   This adjunct taping procedure can be used in conjunction with the basic technique presented.

7

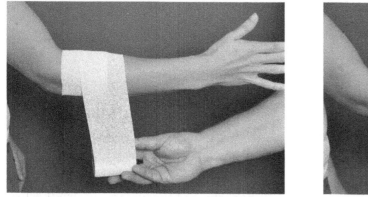

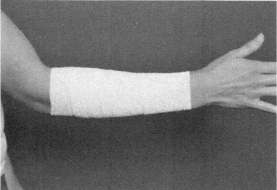

Technique A. Using either 2-in. elastic tape or 3-in. cohesive tape, or elastic wrap, apply a compression technique over the forearm area.

Wrist

Purpose:	To provide support and stability for the wrist
Clinical Application:	Sprains and strains
Anatomical Structure:	Dorsal and palmar radiocarpal ligaments
Anatomical Position:	• Hyperextension: Wrist positioned in slight flexion and fingers spread apart • Hyperflexion: Wrist positioned in slight extension and fingers spread apart
Supplies:	1-in. and 1½-in. adhesive tape and 1-in. and 2-in. elastic tape
Pre-Taping Procedures:	With the wrist in a supinated position, in slight extension and fingers spread apart

Taping Procedures:

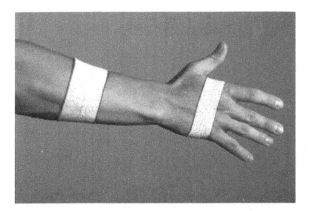

1. Apply two anchor strips of 1-in. and 2-in. elastic tape. Apply the 2-in. anchor around the mid-forearm and the 1-in. anchor around the second through fifth metacarpal heads.

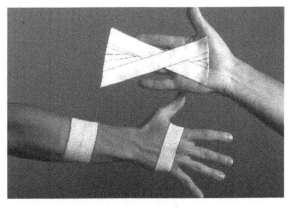

2. Using adhesive tape, construct a five- to seven-strip butterfly pattern that will extend from the proximal anchor to the distal anchor. To prevent hyperflexion, place this butterfly pattern on the dorsal aspect of the hand. To prevent hyperextension, place the butterfly pattern on the palmar aspect of the hand.

7

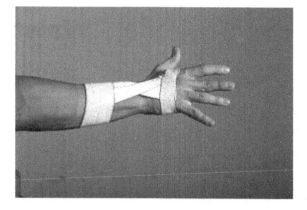

3. Apply a second series of anchor strips.

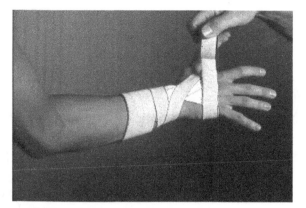

4. Apply a 1-in. strip of elastic tape in a figure of eight pattern. Begin on the dorsal aspect of the forearm, cross diagonally to the second metacarpal, encircle the distal aspect of the second through fifth metacarpals, continue across the palmar aspect to the fifth metacarpal, and cross diagonally to the radial aspect of the wrist and encircle the wrist. Apply two to three figures of eight.

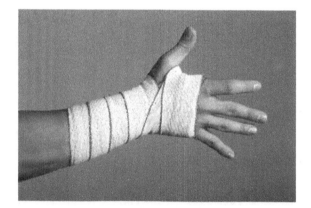

7

5. Apply a final continuous closure strip with 2-in. elastic tape. Begin on the proximal anchor and spiral the tape, overlapping one half of its width, and end on the distal anchor. Secure the elastic tape ends with anchors of adhesive tape.

*Upon completion of the procedure, make sure you check for neatness and gaps, adequate support, along with proper function of the affected area. In certain situations, the individual might be asked to perform function tests to establish appropriate technique application.

Adjunct Taping Procedures: Wrist

This adjunct taping procedure can be used in conjunction with the basic technique presented.

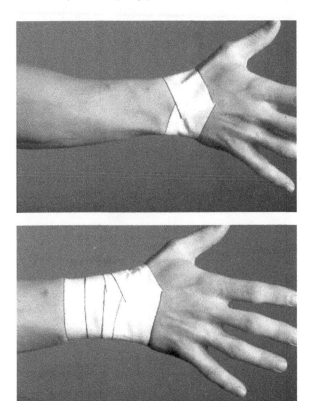

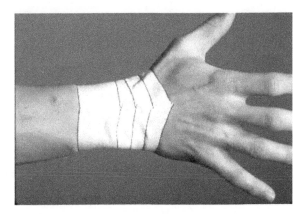

Technique A. In certain sporting activities, tape should not be applied to the palm of the hand. In such situations, apply two layers of four support strips. Begin proximally and work distally. Apply the 1½-in. adhesive tape around the wrist starting at the ulnar styloid process, cross the dorsal aspect of the distal forearm, and encircle the wrist. Overlap the tape by one half of its width each time. Apply the second layer proximally to distally and cover the same area.

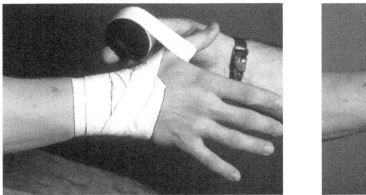

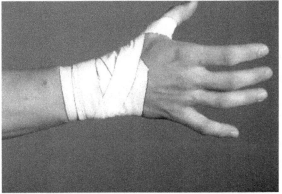

7

Technique B. In conjunction with Technique A, include a thumb spica taping procedure. Starting at the ulnar styloid process, cross the dorsum of the hand, cover the lateral joint line, encircle the thumb, proceed across the palmar aspect of the hand, and finish at the ulnar styloid process.

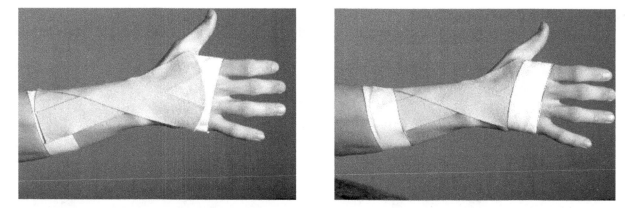

Technique C. Use adhesive felt in place of the adhesive tape butterfly pattern.

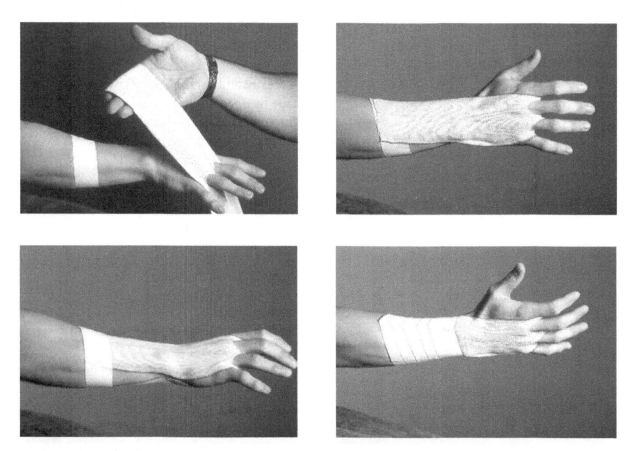

Technique D. Apply an anchor strip of 1½-in. adhesive tape around the mid-forearm. Using 3-in. elastic tape, cut a strip 12 in. to 16 in. in length. In the middle of the tape strip, cut two small holes, approximately 1 in. from each side of the tape. With full tension applied to the tape, place the third and fourth phalanges through the cutouts. Attach the ends of the elastic tape to the mid-forearm anchor. Secure the procedure by applying an anchor of 1½-in. adhesive tape over the tape ends.

Thumb Spica

Purpose:	To provide support and stability for the first metacarpophalangeal (MP) joint of the hand
Clinical Application:	Sprain
Anatomical Structure:	Thumb and wrist
Anatomical Position:	Hand in palm-down position, with thumb slightly flexed and phalanges adducted
Supplies:	1-in. adhesive tape
Pre-Taping Procedures:	With the wrist in a supinated position, in slight extension and fingers spread apart

Taping Procedures:

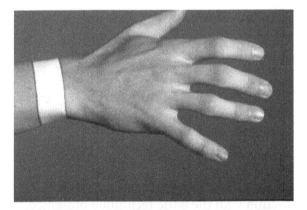

1. Apply an anchor strip of adhesive tape around the wrist. Start at the ulnar styloid process, cross the dorsal aspect of the distal forearm, and encircle the wrist.

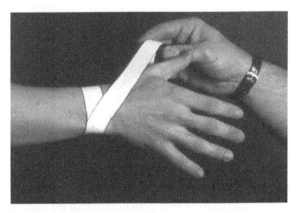

2. Apply the first of three support strips for the first MP joint. Starting at the ulnar styloid process, cross the dorsum of the hand, cover the lateral joint line, encircle the thumb, proceed across the palmar aspect of the hand, and finish at the ulnar condyle.

7

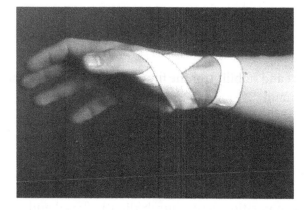

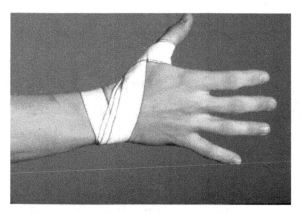

3. This is commonly referred to as a thumb spica. Repeat this procedure.

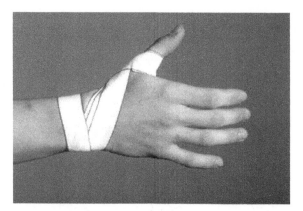

4. To help hold this procedure in place, apply a final anchor strip around the wrist. Check for circulation/skin color at the distal phalanx once you complete the tape procedure.

*Upon completion of the procedure, make sure you check for neatness and gaps, adequate support, along with proper function of the affected area. In certain situations, the individual might be asked to perform function tests to establish appropriate technique application.

Adjunct Taping Procedures: Thumb Spica

    This adjunct taping procedure can be used in conjunction with the basic technique presented.

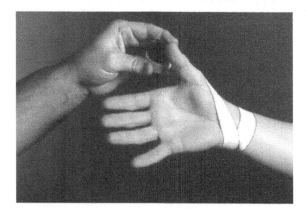

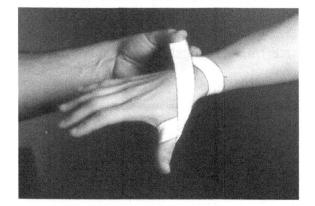

Technique A. In another application of the thumb spica, apply tape in the opposite direction. Apply the first of three support strips for the first MP joint. Starting at the ulnar styloid process, cross the palmar portion of the hand, cover the medial joint line, encircle the thumb, proceed across the dorsum aspect of the hand, and finish at the ulnar styloid process. When you are taping to support the ulnar collateral ligament, this technique may be preferred.

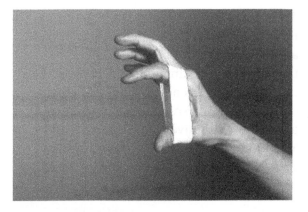
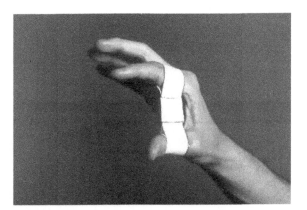

Technique B. Apply thumb c-lock for additional support.

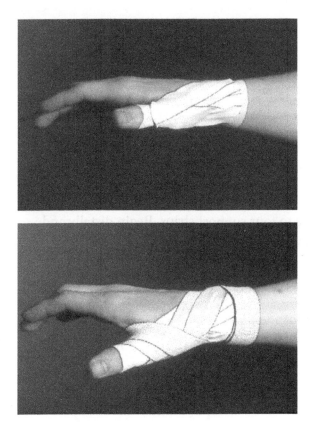

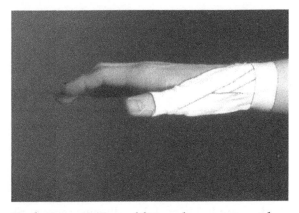

Technique C. For additional support, apply adduction strips. Apply these strips from the dorsal aspect of hand across the thumb and end on palmar surface of the hand. Overlap the tape one half of its width until the first IP joint is covered.

7

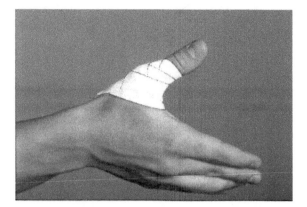

Technique D. Use adhesive tape to form a fan shape (apply four to six strips to provide adequate support). Place the fan-shaped tape from the proximal phalange, cover the affected area, and end on the radial aspect of the wrist. Adhesive felt can be used in place of the adhesive tape. To secure, apply a continuous strip of elastic tape around the thumb and wrist. This joint spica will provide additional support.

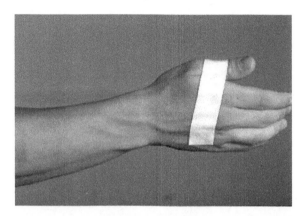
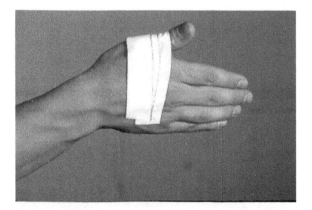

Technique E. Using 1-in. adhesive tape, apply three to four support strips. Begin distally and work proximally. Each strip will resemble a half figure of eight pattern.

7

Finger Splint

Purpose:	To aid in support of the injured interphalangeal (IP) joint
Clinical Application:	General conditions procedure used for sprains to the phalanges of the hand
Anatomical Structure:	Interphalangeal joint
Anatomical Position:	Phalanges placed in extension
Supplies:	½-in. adhesive tape and gauze, felt, or foam rubber
Pre-Taping Procedures:	Cut the gauze to the appropriate size before you begin. Place the phalanges in extension.

Taping Procedures:

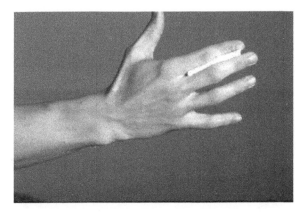

1. Place gauze between affected and adjacent phalanges.

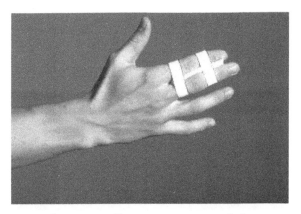

2. Apply ½-in. adhesive tape around the proximal and distal aspects of the affected and adjacent phalanges. This technique is known as buddy taping. In high-risk sports, pair and tape the second and third phalanges and the fourth and fifth phalanges together.

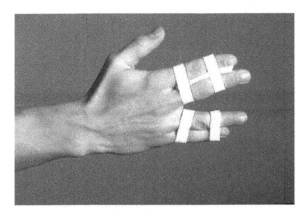

*Upon completion of the procedure, make sure you check for neatness and gaps, adequate support, along with proper function of the affected area. In certain situations, the individual might be asked to perform function tests to establish appropriate technique application.

7

Collateral Interphalangeal Joint

Purpose:	To provide support and stability to the proximal interphalangeal (PIP) joint of the phalanges
Clinical Application:	Sprain to PIP joint
Anatomical Structure:	Interphalangeal joints
Anatomical Position:	With the palmar side of the hand up, phalanges slightly flexed and abducted
Supplies:	½-in. adhesive tape
Pre-Taping Procedures:	Slightly flex the PIP joint

Taping Procedures:

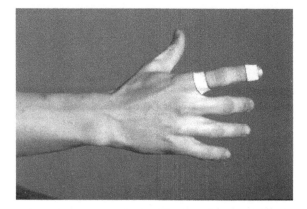

1. Apply anchor strips around proximal and distal aspects of phalanges.

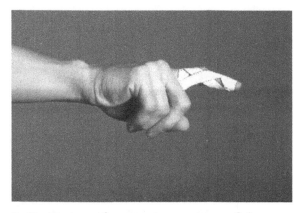

2. Starting on the anterior portion of the proximal anchor, apply the tape, crossing the lateral joint line, going under the finger, and ending on the distal anchor.

7

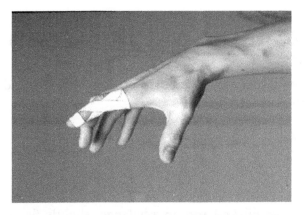

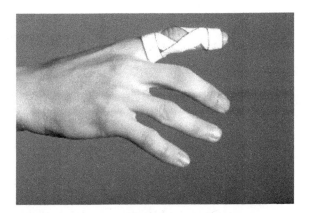

3. Start on the anterior portion of the distal anchor, apply the tape crossing the medial joint line, under the finger, and ending on the proximal anchor.

4. To secure this technique, apply a second anchor over the tape ends. For additional support and to allow greater mobility of the affected joint, this technique can be combined with finger splinting.

*Upon completion of the procedure, make sure you check for neatness and gaps, adequate support, along with proper function of the affected area. In certain situations, the individual might be asked to perform function tests to establish appropriate technique application.

7

Hyperextension of Phalanges

Purpose:	To reduce hyperextension movement of interphalangeal (IP) and metacarpophalangeal (MP) joints
Clinical Application:	Sprains and strains
Anatomical Structure:	Phalanges and hand
Anatomical Position:	With the palmar side of the hand up, phalanges slightly flexed and abducted
Supplies:	½-in. or 1-in. adhesive tape
Pre-Taping Procedures:	Slightly flex the PIP and DIP joints

Taping Procedures:

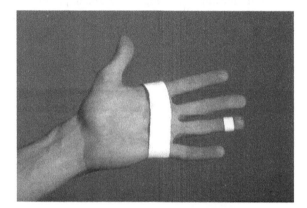

1. Apply an anchor strip around the distal aspect of the second through fifth metacarpals and a second anchor around the distal portion of the affected phalange.

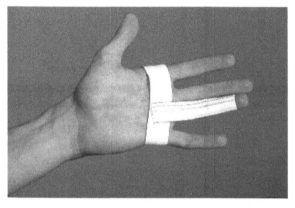

2. Apply two to three stabilizing bars of tape from the proximal anchor to distal anchor on the palmar aspect of the hand.

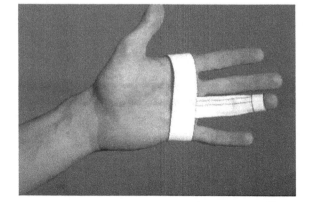

7

3. To secure this technique, apply a second anchor over the original anchors.

*Upon completion of the procedure, make sure you check for neatness and gaps, adequate support, along with proper function of the affected area. In certain situations, the individual might be asked to perform function tests to establish appropriate technique application.

Adjunct Taping Procedures: Hyperextension of Phalanges
This adjunct taping procedure can be used in conjunction with the basic technique presented.

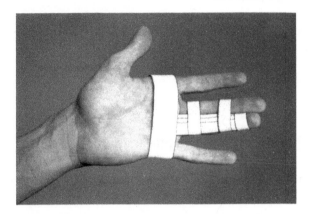

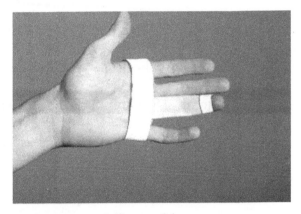

Technique A. For additional support, combine this technique with finger splinting (buddy taping), which will allow greater mobility of the affected joint.

Technique B. Adhesive felt, cut to an appropriate size, can be used as stabilizing bars in place of adhesive tape.

7

Contusion to Hand

Purpose:	To provide protection to the bruised hand
Clinical Application:	Contusions
Anatomical Structure:	Hand and wrist
Anatomical Position:	Palmar aspect of the hand down and phalanges abducted
Supplies:	1-in. and ½-in. adhesive tape, 2-in. elastic tape, and felt or foam pad
Pre-Taping Procedures:	Cut the foam pad before beginning the procedure

Taping Procedures:

7

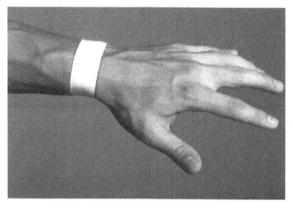

1. Apply an anchor strip of 1-in. adhesive tape around the wrist. Start at the ulnar condyle, cross the dorsal aspect of the distal forearm, and encircle the wrist.

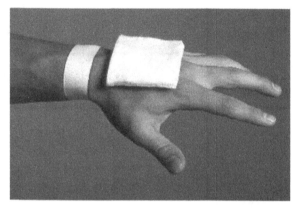

2. Apply the foam pad over the affected area of the hand.

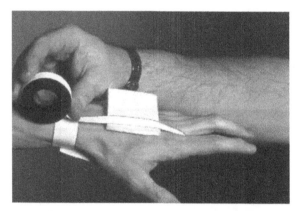

3. Apply strips of ½-in. tape. Start on the palmar aspect of the anchor strip, cross between the phalanges, and end on the dorsal aspect of the anchor strip.

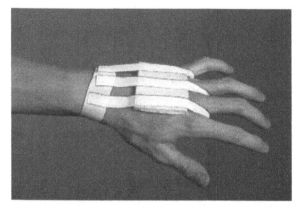

4. Apply three strips, between the second and third, third and fourth, and fourth and fifth phalanges.

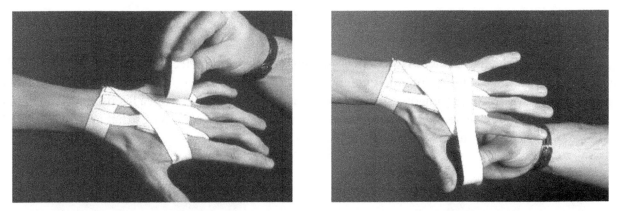

5. Apply a strip of 1-in. adhesive tape in a figure of eight pattern. Begin on the dorsal aspect of the wrist near the ulnar condyle, cross diagonally to the second metacarpal, and encircle the distal aspect of the second through fifth metacarpals. Continue across the palmar aspect to the fifth metacarpal, crossing diagonally to the radial aspect of the wrist and encircling the wrist.

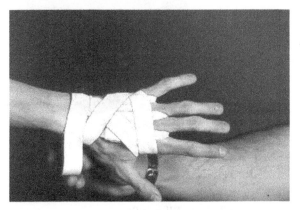

6. Apply two to three figure of eights. Complete this technique by applying a second anchor strip of 1-in. adhesive tape around the wrist.

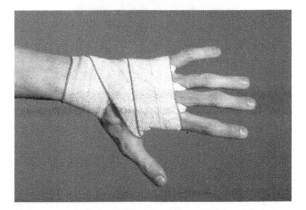

7. Apply a continuous figure of eight strip of 2-in. elastic tape for additional support.

*Upon completion of the procedure, make sure you check for neatness and gaps, adequate support, along with proper function of the affected area. In certain situations, the individual might be asked to perform function tests to establish appropriate technique application.

7

Protective Devices

The use of protective devices is beneficial if they are properly selected, used in the appropriate setting, correctly fitted, and follow the guidelines of the specific sport. Consultation with a medical equipment specialist is highly encouraged! In some cases, a prescription from a licensed physician may result in insurance reimbursement. Listed below are various protective devices that are commercially available in use in sport and/or physical actitivity.

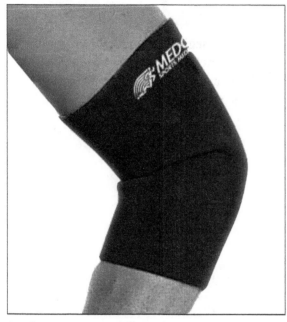

Medco Neoprene Elbow Support

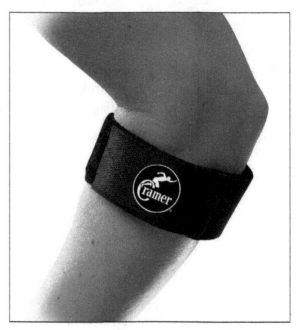

Cramer Tennis Elbow Strap

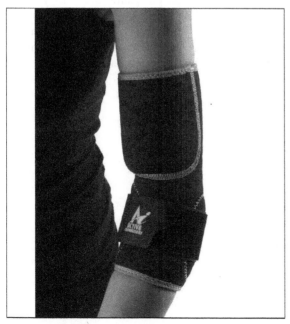

Cramer TBS Elbow Support

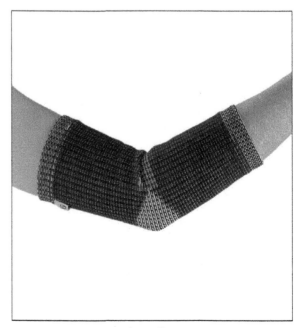

Stromgren Nano Flex Elbow Support

7

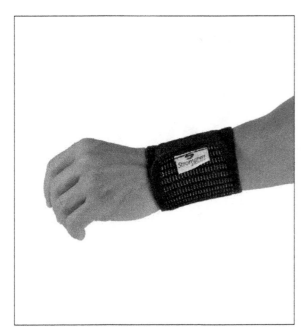

Stromgren Nano Flex Wrist

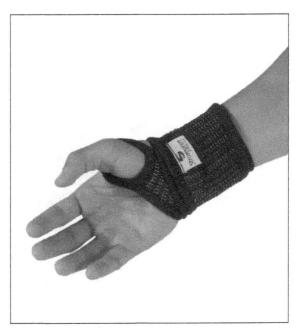

Stromgren Nano Flex Wrist and Thumb

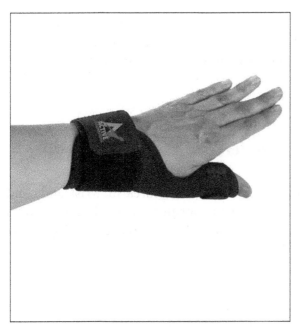

Cramer Moldable Thumb Spica

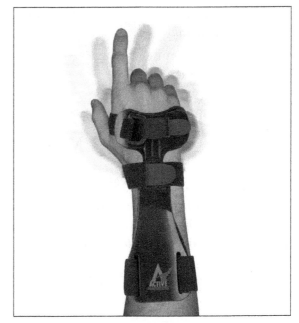

Cramer Dynamic Wrist Orthosis

7

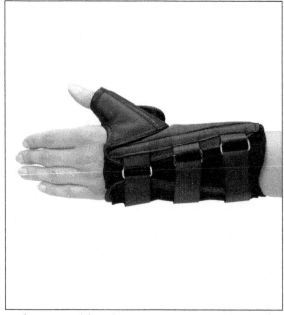

Rolyan Workhard D Ring Wrist and Thumb Support

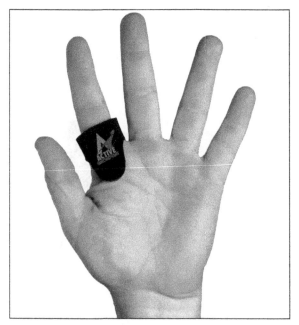

Cramer Digit Cushion

Listed below are various protective devices avilable to use in sport. Because a variety of protective devices are available, a qualified physician or qualified health care professional and medical equipment specialist can determine whether the individual is best suited for an off-the-shelf or custom brace.

- Elbow pad/brace
- Olecranon pad
- Sports compression sleeve

Musculoskeletal Disorders

The following is a list of common musculoskeletal disorders of the elbow, forearm, wrist, and hand. For definitions of these terms, the authors encourage the learner to consult these medical references: *Taber's Medical Dictionary*, *Stedman's Medical Dictionary for the Health Professions and Nursing*, and/or *Signs and Symptoms of Athletic Injuries* (listed in Appendix B).

7

Elbow, Forearm, Wrist, and Hand

Contusion	Wrist and hand
Dislocation	Bontonniere deformity
Epicondylitis	Carpal tunnel syndrome
Forearm splints	De Quervain's tenosynovitis
Hyperextension	Dislocation
Nerve injury	Mallet finger
Olecranon bursitis	Subungual hematoma
Sprain	Sprain
Tendonopathies of elbow	Strain
Ulna nerve contusion	

Part V

Recommendations for Selected Protective Devices

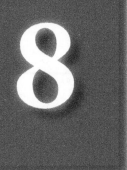

8 Facial, Thorax, Abdomen, and Low Back

Educational Objectives

Upon completing this chapter, the reader will be able to do the following:
- Explain the purpose for a protective device
- Develop skills in the selection of and fit of proper protective devices for specific anatomical structures
- Identify the athletic governing bodies for standards and protection
- Describe and demonstrate the purposes, clinical applications, anatomical structures, supplies needed, and pre-taping and taping procedures for the ribs and low back

Introduction and Disclaimer

The procedures in this text are based on current research and recommendations from professionals in sport medicine and related health care professions. The information is intended to supplement, not substitute, recommendations from a qualified physician, qualified health care professional, and medical equipment specialist. Sagamore Publishing LLC and the authors disclaim responsibility for any adverse effect or consequences resulting from the misapplication or injudicious use of the material contained in the text. It is also accepted as judicious that health care professionals, sport industry professionals, and students must work under the guidance of a qualified physician, qualified health care provider, and medical equipment specialist.

Proper Assessment of Injury

Before applying a preventive technique (tape, wrap, and/or device), a qualified physician or qualified health care professional should complete a proper injury evaluation. Following the injury evaluation, a qualified health care professional and a medical equipment specialist can then recommend a proper protective device. This ensures that the proper device is applied for protection, support, stability, and compression. Also, developing a thorough knowledge of protective devices is imperative for health care professionals.

Terminology

Flexion-the act of bending or condition of being bent in contrast to extension; decrease in the angle between the bones forming a joint.

Extension-a movement that pulls apart both ends of any part; the act of drawing a body segment toward a straight line position with its proximally conjoined body segment, or away from the body joint.

Rotation-process of turning on an axis; movement around a longitudinal axis which passes through a joint as in turning the palm of the hand up or down with the arm abducted.

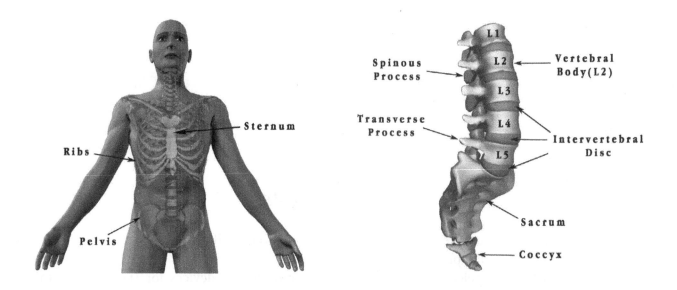

Figure 8.1. Anatomy: Facial, Thorax, Abodomen, and Low Back

Protective Devices

The primary purpose for a protective device is to prevent an injury and to protect injured anatomical structures from further aggravation. Through proper application, a protective device can be applied for additional protection, support, stability, and compression. The use of a protective device can be highly beneficial to the particular body part if properly selected. To avoid violating the manufacturer's specifications, follow suggested guidelines for proper selection, application, and maintenance. A protective device is a commercial product that is well designed and provides manufacturing liability and proper application instructions. The protective device is worn for protection, support, stability, or compression of an anatomical body part. To ensure safety and product effectiveness, the protective device should have product liability coverage from the manufacturer and instructions for proper application. There are sport-specific regulations, rules, and warnings concerning proper athletic equipment. Sport-specific equipment is worn as a standard uniform for participation in order to address the individual's safety. Standards of protection have improved through the combined efforts of athletic governing bodies, the American Society for Testing and Materials (ASTM), the National Operating Committee on Standards for Athletic Equipment (NOCSAE), and the Hockey Equipment Certification Council (HECC).

Medical Device Authorization

As required, a qualified physician or qualified health care professional must prescribe a custom brace. Upon their recommendations, an individual can work with a qualified health care professional and medical equipment specialist for a recommended custom brace. In some cases, a prescription from a licensed physician may result in insurance reimbursement. Figure 8.2 is an example of a "Medical Device Authorization Form."

MEDCO
SPORTS MEDICINE

PRESCRIPTION DRUG & MEDICAL DEVICE
AUTHORIZATION FORM

If purchasing prescription pharmaceuticals, please complete sections A & B
If purchasing an Automated External Defibrillator (AED) unit or other medical device, please complete sections A & C

Dear Valued Customer,

In order to ship you prescription pharmaceuticals and/or medical devices, we must have authorization from a licensed physician or other authorized prescriber. This individual needs to fill out the form below and fax a copy of this page and a photocopy of their license to 800-222-1934.

If your School/Facility does not have a licensed physician or other authorized prescriber, but is licensed to purchase prescription pharmaceuticals and/or medical devices, please fax a copy of the license and this form for identification to 800-222-1934.

A) Name of School/Facility: _____

Attention:_____Customer #:_____

Address: _____

City & State:_____Zip:_____

Phone:_____Fax:_____

E-Mail:_____

B) I hereby authorize the internally designated representatives named below to order prescription products for this School/Facility. (please print)

1._____2._____

Type of authorization: ❑ Unlimited ❑ Limited (please attach list of products)

Physician/Authorized Prescriber Signature: _____

Physician/Authorized Prescriber Name (please print): _____

State License Number: _____
(please include photocopy of license)

C) I hereby acknowledge that I am aware that medical devices are intended for use by a physician or a person certified or trained to use such device.

Name (please print):_____

Title: _____

State License/Certification Number:_____

Signature:_____Date:_____

Call 1-800-55MEDCO   www.medco-athletics.com   Fax 1-800-222-1934   **MEDCO** *SPORTS MEDICINE*   **137**

Figure 8.2. Medco Sports Medicine Prescription Drug and Medical Device Authorization Form

Protective Devices

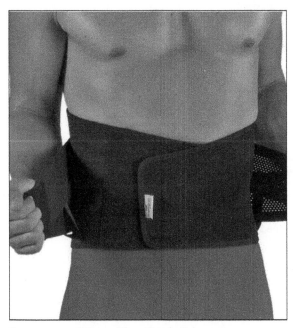

Stromgren Nano Flex Back Support

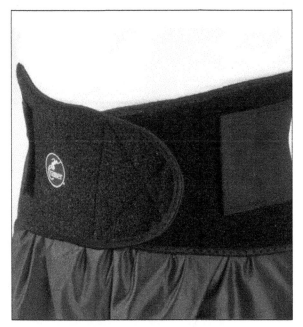

Cramer Lumbar Support

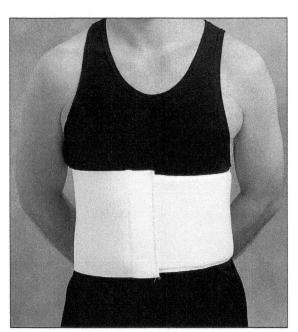

Rolyan Universal Rib Support

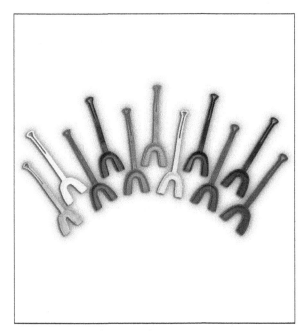

Cramer Mouth Guards

8

Listed below are various protective devices available to use in sport. Because a variety of protective devices are available, a qualified physician or qualified health care professional and medical equipment specialist can determine whether the individual is best suited for an off-the-shelf or custom brace.

- Ear plugs
- Hip pointer brace/guard
- Nose guard
- Sports compression girdle
- Throat protector that attaches for face mask

Taping Techniques

The taping techniques presented are the fundamental procedures. A strong knowledge of anatomy, physiology, and biomechanics is essential. Developing a thorough knowledge regarding the fundamentals about the application of taping/wrapping procedures is imperative. Review Chapter 1 before applying any technique.

Rib.

Purpose:	To provide support and compression to the ribs
Clinical Application:	Contusion and strains
Anatomical Structure:	Thoracic cavity
Anatomical Position:	Standing upright, the arm on the affect side abducted
Supplies:	1½-in. adhesive tape, 4-in. or 6-in. extra long elastic wrap, gauze pad or large Band-Aid, and 2-in. or 3-in. elastic tape

Pre-Taping Procedure:

Taping Procedures:

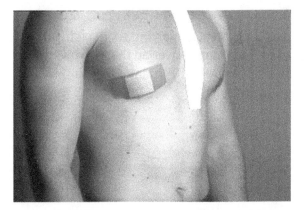

Cover the nipple with either gauze pad or a Band-Aid.

1. On the uninjured side, apply two vertical anchor strips near the anterior and posterior midline of the body. Advise the individual to inhale and expand thorax cavity.

8

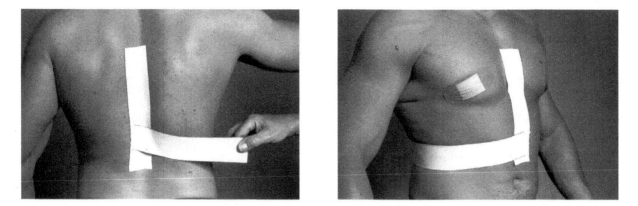

2. Begin with a strip of adhesive tape on the distal aspect of the posterior anchor, follow the contour of the ribs, and end on the distal aspect of the anterior anchor. When applying the tape, have the person inhale.

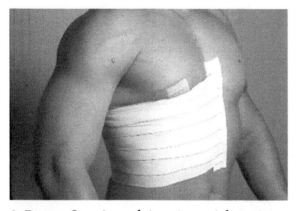

3. Repeat Step 2, applying six to eight strips of adhesive tape. Overlap the tape by one half of its width. Begin interiorly and work superiorly.

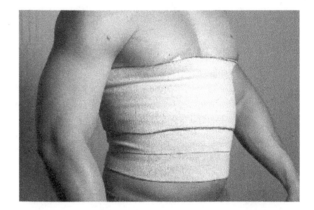

4. Apply a 4-in. or 6-in. extra long elastic wrap over the top. With the person's chest expanded, apply the wrap in a circular manner around the torso, beginning interiorly and working superiorly.

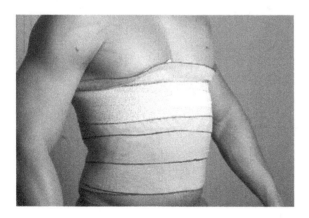

5. Secure the wrap with a continuous strip of elastic tape. Anchor the elastic tape with adhesive tape.

*Upon completion of the procedure, make sure you check for neatness and gaps, adequate support, along with proper function of the affected area. In certain situations, the individual might be asked to perform function tests to establish appropriate technique application.

8

Adjunct Taping Procedures: Rib

These adjunct taping procedures can be used in conjunction with the basic technique presented.

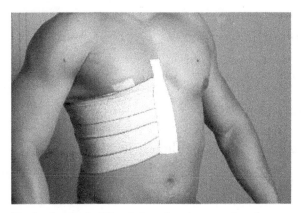

Technique A. Use 3-in. elastic tape in place of the adhesive tape.

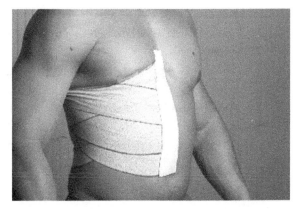

Technique B: The "X" Pattern Technique. Apply the X pattern technique. Begin at the distal aspect of one anchor, cross the affected area, and end on the opposite anchor. Apply the second strip in the same pattern beginning from the opposite anchor. Repeat step 2, three to five times, overlapping the tape by one half of its width.

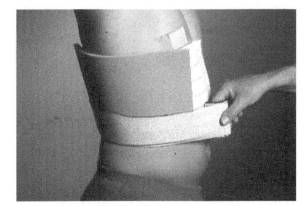

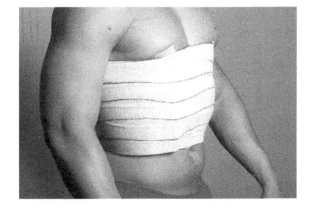

Technique C. Use foam rubber to pad the affected area for additional protection and then secure with elastic tape or elastic wrap.

8

Low Back

Purpose:	To provide support to the low back
Clinical Application:	Sprains, strains, and contusions
Anatomical Structure:	Low back (lumbar and sacral)
Anatomical Position:	Standing position, knees and waist slightly flexed
Supplies:	1½-in. or 2-in. adhesive tape and 6-in. extra long elastic wrap

Taping Procedures:

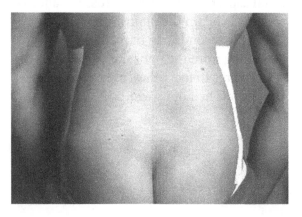

1. Apply two vertical anchor strips, approximately 4 in. to 6 in. in length, over the lateral sides of the torso.

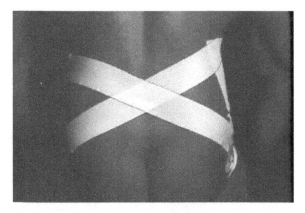

2. Apply the X pattern technique. Begin at the distal aspect of one anchor, cross the affected area, and end on the opposite anchor. Apply the second strip in the same pattern beginning from the opposite anchor.

8

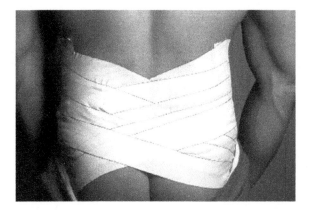

3. Repeat Step 2, seven to nine times, overlapping the tape by one half of its width.

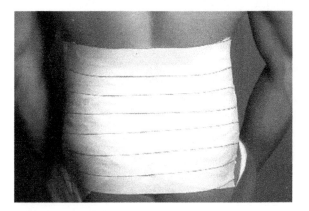

4. Apply parallel strips, working inferior to superior, until the affected area is covered. Overlap each strip by one half of its width. Place a final anchor over each original anchor to help hold the tape in place.

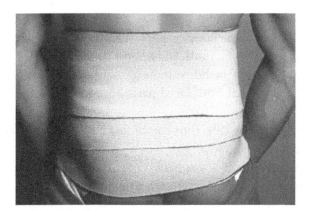

5. Have the individual exhale to expand the abdominal cavity. In a circular fashion, apply the elastic wrap around the waist. Secure the wrap with a strip of adhesive tape.

*Upon completion of the procedure, make sure you check for neatness and gaps, adequate support, along with proper function of the affected area. In certain situations, the individual might be asked to perform function tests to establish appropriate technique application.

Musculoskeletal Disorders

8

The following is a list of common musculoskeletal disorders of the facial, thorax, abdomen, and low back. For definitions of these terms, the authors encourage the learner to consult these medical references: *Taber's Medical Dictionary*, *Stedman's Medical Dictionary for the Health Professions and Nursing*, and/or *Signs and Symptoms of Athletic Injuries* (listed in Appendix B).

Facial, Thorax, Abdomen, and Low Back
Contusion
Sprain
Strain

Appendix A: Glossary

A

Abduction. Lateral movement of a limb away from the median plane of the body; movement away from the median plane around an anterior-posterior axis with the angle between the displaced parts becoming greater, as in lifting the arm sideward away from the body.

Achilles tendon. The tendon of insertion of the gastrocnemius and soleus muscles on the calcaneus; one of the strongest tendons in the body.

Acromioclavicular joint (AC). A gliding or plane joint between the acromion and the acromial end of the clavicle; sprain to joint is known as separate shoulder.

Action. In physiology, the motions or functions of a part or organ of the body.

Acute. Of pain, sharp, severe; of disease, having rapid onset, severe symptoms, and a short course.

Adduction. Lateral movement of a limb toward the median plane of the body; movement toward the median plane around an anterior–posterior axis with the angle between the displaced parts becoming lesser, as in bringing the arm sideward against the body.

Adhesive felt (moleskin). Material contains an adhesive mass on one side, thus combining a cushioning effect with the ability to be held in a specific spot by the adhesive mass.

Adhesive (tape) mass. Adhesive applied to the cloth comprised of natural synthetic, zinc oxide, and so forth.

Anatomical position. The position assumed when a person is standing erect with arms at the sides, palms forward; the neutral stance of the individual.

Anatomical snuffbox. A depression in the skin formed at the posterior base of the thumb when the thumb is extended from the hand; the space at the base of the thumb created by the extensor pollicis longus and brevis tendons.

Anchor. Anything that makes stable or secure, anything that is depended upon for support or security.

Antalgic gait. A gait in which the patient experiences pain during the stance phase and thus remains on the painful leg for as short a time as possible.

Anterior. Before; in front of; in anatomical nomenclature, it refers to the ventral or abdominal side of the body; the front of the body or body part.

Anterior cruciate ligament (ACL). A ligament crossing through the knee joint that attaches from the anterior tibia to the posterior femur. It limits anterior movement of the tibia from the femur, as well as rotation of the tibia.

Appendicular skeleton. The bones that make up the shoulder girdle, upper extremities, pelvis, and lower extremities; these bones form the appendages and attach to the axial skeleton.

Arch. An anatomical structure having a curved or bowlike outline.

Articular surfaces. The ends of bones which move on each other; these surfaces are covered with a thin layer of cartilage (hyaline cartilage) to ensure smooth movement.

Articulation. A joint; the site of close approximation of two or more bones; the manner of connecting by a joint.

Avascular. Lacking in blood vessels or having a poor blood supply, said of tissues such as cartilage.

Avulsion. A tearing away forcibly of a part or structure.

Axial skeleton. Composed of the bones of the skull, the thorax, and the vertebral column. These bones form the axis of the body.

Axilla. Armpit.

B

Base strip. Supportive strips to taping procedure.

Biceps. The muscle of the upper arm that flexes the elbow and supinates the forearm; muscle on front of upper arm.

Bloodborne pathogens. Bloodborne pathogens are infectious microorganisms in human blood that can cause disease in humans. These pathogens include, but are not limited to, hepatitis B (HBV), hepatitis C (HCV) and human immunodeficiency virus (HIV). Needlesticks and other sharps-related injuries may expose workers to bloodborne pathogens. Workers in many occupations, including first aid team members, housekeeping personnel in some industries, nurses and other health care personnel may be at risk of exposure to bloodborne pathogens.

Bone. A supportive rigid connective tissue consisting of an abundant calcified matrix enclosing many branched cells.

Brace. Any one of a great variety of devices used in orthopedics for increasing stability of joints or extremities.

Buckle. A fastening device for two loose ends that is attached to one and holds the other by a catch.

Bunion. Inflammation and thickening of the first metatarsal joint of the great toe, usually associated with marked enlargement of the joint and lateral displacement of the toe

Bursa. A fluid-filled sac or saclike cavity that allows a muscle or tendon to slide over bone (thereby eliminating friction). *Bursae* means plural.

Bursitis. Inflammation of a bursa, especially between bony prominences and muscle or tendon, as in the shoulder and knee. It is typically caused by repeated stresses placed on a joint during work or play, but sometimes results from sudden trauma, from inflammatory joint disease, or bacteria. Common forms include rotator cuff, miner's or tennis elbow, and prepatellar bursitis.

Butterfly. Strips of tape that overlap in an X pattern; an adhesive bandage used in place of sutures to hold wound edges together.

C

Calcaneus. The heel bone; it articulates with the cuboid bone and with the talus.

Cantilever. Shapes and supports the arch; spreads force to front and rear of shell on flat or noncantilever pads.

Cap or Cup. Shoulder pad padding that covers deltoid/humerus.

Cartilage. A connective tissue characterized by its nonvascularity and firm consistency.

Cast. To produce a specific form by pouring material (metal, plaster, etc.) into a prepared mold; used to immobilize an anatomical body part.

Cervical. Pertaining to or in the region of the neck; seven vertebrae in the neck.

Check rein. Reinforced tape to prevent movement; restricts range of motion.

Chondral. Pertaining to cartilage.

Chrondromalacia patella. Chondromalacia at the front of the knee, accompanied by pain and crepitus, and often affecting younger athletes.

Chronic. Of long duration; long lasting; persistent.

Circumduction. Movement around an axis such that the proximal end of a limb is fixed and the distal end traces a circle.

Clavicle channel. Shoulder pad padding that is structured in such a way to provide a gap between the pad and the AC joint.

Closed cell foam. Material that is firm and is one layer, retains its shape quickly.

Close out strips. Final strips of adhesive or elastic tape that are applied to finalize taping procedure; usually applied distal to proximal.

Coccyx. A small bone at the base of the spinal column in humans, formed by four fused rudimentary vertebrae; it is usually ankylosed and articulated with the sacrum above.

Cohesive bandage (wrap and/or tape). A bandage made of material that sticks to itself but not to other substances, used to bandage fingers and extremities or to build up pads.

Collateral. Accompanying; side-by-side (i.e., medial and lateral).

Collateral ligament. A ligament that provides medial and lateral stability to joints, including the medial (ulnar) and lateral (radial) collateral ligaments at the elbow, the medial (tibial) and lateral (fibular) collateral ligaments at the knee, the medial (deltoid) and lateral collateral ligaments at the ankle, and the collateral ligaments of the fingers.

Compression. The act of applying pressure to a body part (i.e., applying an elastic wrap: begin the elastic wrap distally, farthest from the heart; cover the injury; and spiral the wrap toward the heart on the involved anatomical structure).

Condyle. A rounded protuberance at the end of a bone forming an articulation.

Contract. To draw together, reduce in size, or shorten.

Contusion. Compression to anatomical structure; injury caused by direct contact.

Costochondral. Pertaining to the rib and its cartilage.

Cotton. A soft, white, fibrous material obtained from the fibers enclosing the seeds of various plants of the Malvaceae, especially those of the genus *Gossypium*; the ability to absorb, to hold emollients, and to offer a mild padding effect.

Cover strip or bandage. A piece of soft, usually absorbent gauze or other material applied to a limb or other part of the body as a dressing.

Cranial. Pertaining to the cranium.

Cruciate. Cross-shaped, as in the cruciate ligaments of the knee.

Cubital Fossa. Triangular area on the anterior aspect of the forearm directly opposite the elbow joint (the bend of the elbow).

Custom brace. Made to individual specifications and fitted by a qualified health care professional and medical equipment specialist; used to protect specific anatomical structures.

Cutaneous. Pertains to the skin.

D

Depression (down). Just the opposite, as in lowering the shoulder.

Dermal. Pertaining to the dermis; cutaneous.

Dermatome. A band or region of skin supplied by a single sensory nerve.

Diagonally. A slanted or oblique direction.

Diamond shape. An object that is in the shape of two equilateral triangles placed base to base.

Diarthrodial joint. A joint characterized by the presence of a cavity within the capsule separating the bones, permitting considerable freedom of movement; ball and socket joint.

Digit. A finger or toe.

Disinfectant. A substance that prevents infection by killing bacteria.

Dislocation. The displacement of any part, especially the temporary displacement of a bone from its normal position in a joint.

Distal. Farthest from the center, from a medial line, or from the trunk; opposed to proximal.

Distal to proximal. A term commonly used in a taping or wrapping procedure that describes applying material distal (farther away) to proximal (closest); closure strips.

Dorsal. Upper surface (e.g., top of foot).

Dorsiflexion. The act of drawing the toe or foot toward the dorsal aspect of the proximally conjoined body segment; opposite of plantar flexion.

Dorsum. Pertains to the dorsum (back); lying on the back with the face upward; supine; toward the back of an organism.

Dual density foam. Material that has a hard side to disperse the blow and a soft side to absorb impact.

E

Elevation. A raised area that protrudes above the surrounding area; up, as in lifting the shoulder up.

Epaulet. The plastic flap on the shoulder region of shoulder pads, held in place by snubbers; allows movement but returns in place.

Epicondylitis. Inflammation of the epicondyle of the humerus and surrounding tissues.

Epiphysis. A center for ossification at each extremity of long bones; growth plate.

Eversion. Turning outward; the act of rotating the pronated foot externally on the ankle; turning the sole of the foot outward.

Exostosis. A bony growth that arises from the surface of a bone, often involving the ossification of muscular attachments.

Extension. A movement that pulls apart both ends of any part; the act of drawing a body segment toward a straight line position with its proximally conjoined body segment, or away from the body joint.

Exterior or Peripheral. The opposite of interior or internal; near the surface.

External rotation. Turning outwardly or away from the midline of the body.

F

Fascia. A fibrous membrane covering, supporting, and separating tissue; two kinds of fascia: deep fasciae for muscles and superficial fasciae for connecting the skin to the muscles.

Felt. A material composed of matted wool fibers pressed into varying thickness that range from $1/16$ in. to 1 in.

Figure of eight. The bandaging of a joint where the initial turn circles the one part of the joint and the second turn circles the adjoining part of the joint to form a figure of eight (number 8).

Flexion. The act of bending or condition of being bent in contrast to extension; decrease in the angle between the bones forming a joint.

Foam. Material that is made in different thickness and densities that is usually resilient, nonabsorbent, and able to protect the body against compressive forces.

Friction. Rubbing; any force that resists motion that is generated when two surfaces move with respect to each other.

Frontal plane. A flat surface formed by making a cut, imaginary or real, through the body or a part of it. Planes are used as points of reference by which positions of parts of the body are indicated. In the human subject, all planes are based on the body being in an upright anatomical position.

G

Gamekeeper's thumb. An injury to the ulnar collateral ligament of the metacarpophalangeal joint of the thumb.

Gauze. Thin, loosely woven muslin or similar material used for bandages and surgical sponges; assembled in varying thickness and can be used as an absorbent or protective pad.

Glenohumeral joint (GH). Pertaining to the humerus and the glenoid cavity.

H

Hamstrings. Muscle group in the posterior thigh consisting of the semitendinosus, semimembranosus, and biceps femoris.

Heat plastic foam. Plastic that has difference in densities as a result of the addition of liquids, gas, or crystals.

Heel lock. Commonly used in ankle taping, this supportive technique aids in stabilizing the calcaneus.

Hematoma. A swelling comprising a mass of extravasated blood (usually clotted) confined to an organ, tissue, or space and caused by a break in a blood vessel.

Hip pointer. Bruise (contusion) to iliac crest and tissue.

Horizontal plane. A transverse plane at right angles to the vertical axis of the body.

Horizontal strip. A strip of tape or felt tape that is placed horizontal, as opposed to vertical.

Horseshoe. Padding made to resemble a U shape.

Hot spot. Early redness of the skin from friction that could result in a blister formation if preventive measures are not taken.

Hyper. Over, above, excessive.

Hyperextension. Extreme or abnormal extension of a joint, usually the result of trauma, increased muscle tone.

Hyperflexion. Increased flexion of a joint, usually the result of trauma, decreased muscle tone, or joint laxity.

Hypoallergenic. Having diminished potential for causing an allergic reaction.

I

Iliac crest. The anatomical landmark for the superior margin of the pelvis, located between the anterosuperior and posterosuperior iliac spines; a contusion to this area is called a "hip pointer."

Immobilizer. A device to protect and limit the mobility of a specific anatomical body part.

Impingement. Degenerative alteration in a joint in which there is excessive friction between joint tissues; this typically causes limitations in range of motion and the perception of joint pain.

Inferior. Beneath; lower; used medically in reference to the undersurface of an organ or to indicate a structure below another structure.

Insertion. The movable attachment of the distal end of a muscle, which produces shape changes or skeletal movement when the muscle contracts.

Internal. Within the body; within or on the inside; enclosed; inward; the opposite of external.

Internal rotation. Turning inwardly or toward the midline of the body.

Interphalangeal joint (IP). In a joint between two phalanges; in hand and feet, the distal interphalangeal joint (DIP) and proximal interphalangeal joint (PIP).

Inversion. Turning inward; the act of rotating the pronated foot internally on the ankle; turning the sole of the foot inward.

J

Joint capsule. A sheath or continuous enclosure around an organ or structure; a capsula; articular capsule and/or synovial capsule—a saclike, fibrous membrane that surrounds a joint; often including or interwoven with ligaments.

Joint range of motion. The possible excursion of motion at a joint, accomplished by an examiner, without any muscle contraction by the patient. The excursion can be measured by a goniometer and is normally slightly greater than active range of motion. The examiner assesses the maximum excursion at both its beginning and its end; the maximum range of movement of a joint measured in degrees of a circle.

K

Kinesiology. The study of muscles and body movement.

L

Lace. A cord or string used for drawing together two edges such as a garment or shoe.

Lambs wool. A material commonly used on and around the athlete's toes when circular protection is required.

Lateral. Pertains to the side; farther from the midline plane; away from the midline plane.

Lateral epicondylitis (tennis elbow). Tendinitis occurring at the lateral epicondyle; this injury is commonly seen as a result of overuse of the elbow or repetitive wrist extension.

Ligament. A band or sheet of strong fibrous connective tissue connecting the articular ends of bones, binding them together to limit.

Longitudinal arch. The anteroposterior arch of the foot; the medial portion is formed by the calcaneus, talus, navicular, the three cuneiform bones, and the first three metatarsals; the lateral portion is formed by the calcaneus, cuboid, and the fourth and fifth metatarsals.

Lumbar. Pertains to the loins (the part of the back between the thorax and pelvis); vertebral column extending from the 20ᵗʰ through the 24ᵗʰ vertebrae; low back.

M

Major. Means greater or larger.

Malleable. Having the property of being shaped by press.

Malleolus. The protuberance on both sides of the ankle joint; the lower extremity of the fibula is the lateral malleolus and lower end of the tibia is the medial malleolus.

Mechanism of injury. The manner in which a physical injury occurred; the mechanism of injury is used to estimate the forces involved in trauma and thus the potential severity for wounding, fractures, and internal organ damage that a patient may suffer as a result of the injury.

Medial. Pertains to the middle; nearer to the midline plane; toward the midline plane.

Medial epicondylitis (baseball and/or golfers elbow). Tendinitis occurring at the medial epicondyle. This injury is commonly seen as a result of overuse of the elbow or repetitive wrist flexion.

Mallet finger. A flexion deformity of the distal joint of a finger, caused by avulsion of the extensor tendon.

Metacarpophalangeal joint (MCP). Joint between the metacarpus and the phalanges.

Metatarsal arch. The metarsal arch of the foot formed by the metatarsal and proximal bones of the foot.

Memory foam. Material that has varying thickness and slow recovery to impact.

Meniscus. Interarticular fibrocartilage of crescent shape, found in certain joints, especially the lateral and medial menisci (semilunar cartilages) of the knee joint.

Metal grommets. The material that protects/strengthens opening for eyelets.

Midsagittal plane. A vertical plane through the trunk and head dividing the body into right and left halves.

Minor. Of lesser or inferior importance, size, scope, or effect.

Muscle. A type of tissue composed of contractile cells; a contractile organ composed of muscle tissue, affecting the movements of the organs and parts of the body.

Muscle contracted. Active contraction of the muscle by the involved individual.

Myositis ossification. Bone formation occurring at an abnormal anatomical site, usually in soft tissue (e.g., ossification of the intramuscular fascia after an injury).

N

Nerve. Parallel axons running together inside a thick connective tissue sheath (an epineurium); a bundle of nerve fibers, usually outside the brain or spinal cord.

O

Off-the-shelf braces. Brace made in standard sizes and available from merchandise in stock.

Olecrannon. A large process of the ulna projecting behind the elbow joint and forming the bony prominence of the elbow.

Open cell foam. Material that is soft and layered.

Origin. The source of anything; a starting point.

Orthotic. Relating to orthosis; supportive device used for injuries to the foot and ankle.

Overuse syndrome. An injury that results from repetitive use or overuse of a part of the body or from external pressure or environmental conditions that can affect bones, joints bursae, muscles, tendons, nerves, or other anatomical structures.

P

Pad support. A pad placed in a certain area to sustain, hold up, or maintain a desired position.

Palmar. Ventral aspect of the hand; palm of the hand.

Patella. A lens-shaped sesamoid bone situated in front of the knee in the tendon of the quadriceps femoris muscle.

Peroneal tendinitis. Inflammation of the peroneal tendons.

Pes cavus. High arch; deformities of the foot.

Pes planus. Flat feet.

Phalanges. Bones of the fingers (hand) or toes (foot).

Plantar. Pertains to the sole of the foot; ventral aspect.

Plantar fascia. The fascia investing the muscles of the sole of the foot.

Plantar fasciitis. Painful inflammation of the heel and bottom surface of the foot caused by excessive stretching of the fibrous tissue (fascia) that attaches the heel to the forefoot.

Plantar flexion. Extension of the foot so that the forepart is depressed with respect to the position of the ankle; act of drawing the toe or foot toward the plantar aspect of the proximally conjoined body segment; opposite of dorsiflexion.

Plantar (Joplin) neuroma. A compression neuropathy affecting the nerve that supplies sensation to the medial side of the great toe. The condition often occurs in runners or in people whose shoes are too tight at the metatarsophalangeal joint, where the medial plantar proper digital nerve is found.

Popliteal space (fossa). The space behind the knee joint, containing the popliteal artery and vein and small sciatic and popliteal nerves.

Position. The place or arrangement in which something is put; the manner in which a body is arranged for examination.

Posterior. In human anatomy, pertains to or located at or toward the back; dorsal; in human anatomy, *caudal*, *dorsal*, and *posterior* mean the same thing: situated behind.

Posterior cruciate ligament (PCL). A ligament crossing through the knee joint that attaches posteriorly on the tibia and crosses to the inside of the knee on the anterior portion of the medial condyle of the femur.

PRICES. Acronym for protection, rest, ice, compression, elevation, and support.

Pronation. The act of lying prone or facing downward; the act of turning the hand so that the palm faces downward or backward.

Prone. Horizontal with the face downward.

Prophylactic. Any agent or regimen that contributes to the prevention of infection and disease; denoting something that is preventative or protective.

Proprioception. The awareness of posture, movement, and changes in equilibrium and the knowledge of position, weight, and resistance of objects in relation to the body.

Protraction. The extension forward or drawing forward of a part of the body such as the mandible.

Proximal. Nearest the point of attachment, center of the body, or point of reference; the opposite of distal.

Proximal to distal. A term commonly used in taping or wrapping procedure that describes applying material from proximal (closes) to distal (farther away).

Q

Q angle. The acute angle formed by a line from the anterior superior iliac spine of the pelvis through the center of the patella and a line from the tibial tubercle through the patella. The angle describes the tracking of the patella in the trochlear groove of the femur.

Quadriceps. The muscle group in the anterior thigh consisting of the rectus femoris, vastus medialis, vastus intermedius, and vastus lateralis.

R

Range of motion (ROM). The extent to which a body part can move through all of its planes of movement; types of range of motion include active, assistive, passive, and resistive.

Rehabilitation. The processes of treatment and education that help disabled individuals to attain maximum function.

Resilient material. The ability to regain shape after impact; commonly used in areas subject to repeated impact.

Retinaculum. A band or membrane holding any organ or part in its place.

Retraction. The act of drawing backward or the condition of being drawn back; shortening.

Rotary forces. A force generated by active or passive motion that rotates about an axis.

Rotation. Process of turning on an axis; movement around a longitudinal axis which passes through a joint as in turning the palm of the hand up or down with the arm abducted.

Rotator cuff. A musculotendinous structure consisting of supraspinatus, infraspinatus, teres minor, and subscapularis tendons blending with the shoulder joint capsule. The muscles, which surround the glenohumeral joint below the superficial musculature, stabilize and control the head of the humerus in all arm motions, function with the deltoid to abduct the arm, and rotate the humerus.

S

Sagittal plane. A vertical plane through the longitudinal axis of the body or part of the body, dividing it into right and left parts. If it is through the anteroposterior midaxis and divides the body into right and left halves, it is called a *median* or *midsagittal* plane.

Sesamoid bone. A type of short bone occurring in the hands and feet and embedded in tendons or joint capsules.

Sesamoiditis. Inflammation of a sesamoid bone.

Shin splints (medial tibial stress syndrome or medial tibial syndrome). Pain in the anterior, posterior, or posterolateral compartment of the tibia. It usually follows strenuous or repetitive exercise and is often related to faulty foot mechanics such as pes planus or pes cavus. The cause may be ischemia of the muscles in the compartment, minute tears in the tissues, or partial avulsion from the periosteum of the tibial or peroneal muscles. Proper shoes and foot orthotics may help to prevent onset of the condition.

Shoelace. A lace used for fastening shoes or orthopedic devices.

Shorten the angle of pull. Decreasing the range of motion of a joint.

Spica. A figure eight (8) bandage/wrap that generally overlaps the previous to form V-like designs; used to give support, to apply pressure, or to hold a dressing; figure of eight wraps are placed over ankle, knee, elbow, wrist, and hand joints.

Spiral. Applying a bandage around a limb that ascends the body part overlapping the previous bandage.

Sprain. Trauma to ligaments that causes pain and disability depending on the degree of injury to the ligaments.

Stirrup. Any U-shaped loop or piece.

Strain. Trauma to muscles and tendons from violent contraction or excessive or forcible stretch; it may be associated with failure of the synergistic action of muscles.

Strap. To support an injured joint with overlapping strips of adhesive or elastic plaster or tape.

Subluxation. Partial or incomplete dislocation.

Subtalar joint. Any of the three articular surfaces on the inferior surface of the talus.

Superficial. Pertains to or situated near the surface.

Superior. Toward the top of the body or body part.

Supination. The turning of the palm or the hand anteriorly or the foot inward and upward; the act of lying flat upon the back; the condition of being on the back or having the palm of the hand facing upward or the foot turned inward and upward.

Supine. Lying on the back with the face upward; dorsal; a position of the hand or foot with the palm or foot facing upward; the opposite of prone.

Support. To sustain, hold up, or maintain a desired position.

Surface anatomy. The study of the form and markings of the surface of the body, especially as they relate to underlying structures.

Swelling. An abnormal transient enlargement, especially one appearing on the surface of the body. Ice applied to the area helps to limit swelling.

Syndesmosis ankle sprain. Damage to the ligamentous structures of the distal tibiofibular syndesmotic joint, resulting from dorsiflexion or external rotation of the talus within the ankle mortise, or both, which in turn causes spreading of the joint. The distal tibiofibular syndesmosis is formed by the anterior tibiofibular ligament, the interosseous membrane, and the posterior tibiofibular ligament.

T

Tendinitis. Inflammation of a tendon.

Tendon. Fibrous connective tissue serving for the attachment of muscles to bones and other parts.

Tenosynovitis. inflammation of a tendon sheath.

Thenar eminence. A prominence formed by muscles on the palm below the thumb; known as thenar web space

Thoracic. Pertains to the chest or thorax (chest).

Transverse arch. The transverse arch of the foot formed by the navicular, cuboid, cuneiform, and metatarsal bones.

Transverse plane. A horizontal plane at right angles to the vertical axis of the body. A plane that divides the body into a top and bottom portion.

U

Ulnar (medial) collateral ligament (elbow). Ligament that provides medial stability to the elbow joint.

Ulnar collateral ligament (thumb). Ligament that provides medial stability to the thumb joint.

V

Valgus. Bent or turned outward, used especially of deformities in which the most distal anatomical part is angled outward and away from the midline of the body.

Varus. Bent or turned inward, used especially of deformities in which the most distal anatomical part is turned inward and toward the midline of the body.

Ventral. Bottom surface; opposite of dorsal.

Vertical strip. A strip that is placed perpendicular to the line of the horizon, opposed to horizontal strip.

Viscoelastic material. Substance having both viscous and elastic properties.

Volar. Ventral aspect of the hand.

X

X pattern. The crossing of three or more pieces of tape in the shape of a fan.

Appendix B:
Bibliography

American Academy of Orthopedic Surgeons. (1965). *Joint motion: Method of measuring and recording*. New York, NY: Churchill Livingstone.

American Academy of Orthopaedic Surgeons. (2005). *Athletic training and sports medicine*. Chicago, IL: Author.

Anderson, M., & Hall, S. (2012). *Foundations of athletic training*. Baltimore, MD: Lippincott Williams & Wilkins.

Andrews, J., Clancy, W., & Whiteside, J. (1997). *On-field evaluation and treatment of common athletic injuries*. St. Louis, MO: McGraw-Hill Higher Education.

Bachmann, L., Kolb, E., Koller, M., Steurer, J., & Ter Riet, G. (2003). Accuracy of Ottawa ankle rules to exclude fractures of the ankle and mid-foot: A systematic review. British *Medical Journal, 326*(7), 417–419.

Barker, S., Wright, K., & Wright, V. (2001). *Sports injuries 3D* (3rd ed.). Gardner, KS: Cramer Products.

Bartial, D. C., & Campagna, A. J. (1990). Resilient semi-rigid orthopedic support devices. Retrieved from http://www.google.com/patents/US4893617?dq=protective+devices+in+athletics

Beam, J. (2012). *Orthopedic taping, wrapping, bracing and padding* (2nd ed.). Philadelphia, PA: F. A. Davis.

Bicici, S., Karatas, N., & Baltaci, G. (2012). Effect of athletic taping and kinesiotaping on measurements of functional performance in basketball players with chronic inversion ankle sprains. *The International Journal of Sports Physical Therapy, 7*(2), 154–166.

Birkholz, R. D., & Scholz, M. T. (1991). Orthopedic splinting and casting article. Retrieved from http://www.google.com/patents/US5027803?dq=casting+and+splinting

Booher, J., & Thibodeau, G. (2000). *Athletic injury assessment*. St. Louis: McGraw-Hill Higher Education.

Carpenter, T., Easter, D. A., Grim, T. E., Guza, D. E., Hughes, K. E., McGinnis, V., & Whitmore, R. S. (1991). Soft-goods type, formable orthopaedic cast. Retrieved from http://www.google.com/patents/US4996979?dq=casting+and+splinting

Centers for Disease Control and Prevention. (1989). *Guidelines for prevention of transmission of human immunodeficiency virus and hepatitis B virus to health-care and public workers*. Retrieved from http://www.cdc.gov/mmwr/preview/mmwrhtml/0001450.htm

Cerney, J. (1972). *Complete book of athletic taping techniques*. Upper Saddle River, NJ: Prentice Hall.

Cordova, M., Ingersoll, C., & Palieri, R. (2002) Efficacy of prophylactic ankle support: An experimental perspective. *Journal of Athletic Training, 37*(4), 446.

Davis, B. L. (1994). Protective device. Retrieved from http://www.google.com/patents/US5307521?dq=protective+devices+in+athletics

Deere, R., & Wright, K. (2004). Health insurance portability and accountability act: Does it affect you? *KAHPERD Journal, 40*(2), 32.

Deere, R., Wright, K., & Gibson, F. (2003). Open basket taping for acute ankle sprain. *KAHPERD Journal, 39*(1), 26–27.

Deivert, R. (1994). Functional thumb taping procedure. *Journal of Athletic Training, 29*(4), 357.

Des Rochers, D. M., & Cox, D. E. (2002). Proprioceptive benefits derived from ankle support. *Athletic Therapy Today, 7*(6), 44.

Ellis, T. H. (1991). Sports protective equipment. Retrieved from http://europepmc.org/abstract/MED/1788362/reload=2;jsessionid=m031N8JJUtSuxsgaLCma.36

Firer, P. (1990). Effectiveness of taping for the prevention of ankle ligament sprains. *British Journal of Sports Medicine, 24*(1), 47–50.

Fletcher, S., Whitehill, W., & Wright, K. (1993). Medicated compress for blister treatment. *Journal of Athletic Training, 28*(1), 81–82.

Floyd, R. T. (2012). *Manual of structural kinesiology* (18th ed.). New York, NY: McGraw-Hill Higher Education.

France, R. (2011). *Introduction to sports medicine and athletic training* (2nd ed.). New York, NY: Thomson Delmar Learning.

Fratesi, G. R. (1992) Thigh and knee protective device. Retrieved from www.google.com/patents/US5107823?dq=protective+devices+in+athletics

Gallaspy, J., & May, D. (1996). *Signs and symptoms of athletic injuries.* St. Louis, MO: McGraw-Hill Higher Education.

Gehlsen, G. M., Pearson, D., & Bahamonde, R. (1991) Ankle joint strength, total work, and rom: Comparison between prophylactic devices. *Athletic Training Journal, 26*(2), 62–65.

Green, T. A., & Hillman, S. K. (1990). Comparison of support provided by a semiridgid orthosis and adhesive ankle taping before, during, and after exercise. *American Journal of Sports Medicine, 18*(5), 498–506.

Holmes, C., Wilcox, D., & Fletcher, J. (2002). Effect of a modified, low-dye medial longitudinal rch taping procedure on the subtalar joint neutral position before and after light exercise. *Orthpo Sports Physical Therapy, 32*(4), 305–309.

Hoppenfeld, S. (1995). *Physical examination of the spine and extremities.* New York, NY: Appleton-Lang.

Johnson & Johnson. (1986). *Athletic uses of adhesive tape.* Skillman, NJ: Author.

Johnson & Johnson Consumer Products. (1993). *Athletic uses of adhesive tape.* Skillman, NJ: Author.

Kaneko, S., & Takasaki, H. (2011). Forearm pain, diagnosed as intersection syndrome, managed by taping: A case series. *Journal of Orthopaedic & Sports Physical Therapy, 41*(7), 514–519.

Kase, K. (1998). *Kinesio taping perfect manual: Amazing taping therapy to eliminate pain and muscle disorder.* Kinesio Taping Association: Albuquerque, NM.

Kase, K., Wallis, J., & Tsuyoshi, K. (2003). *Clinical therapeutic applications of the kinesio taping method* (2nd ed.). Kinesio Taping Association: Albuquerque, NM.

Knight, K., & Brumels, K. (2009). *Assessing clinical proficiencies in athletic training.* Champaign, IL: Human Kinetics.

Lacroix, V. J. (2000). A complete approach to groin pain. *Physician and Sports Medicine, 28*(1), 66.

Lumbroso, D., Ziv, E., Vered, E., & Kalichman, L. (in press). The effect of Kinesio Tape application on hamstring and gastrocnemius muscles in healthy young adults. *Journal of Bodywork & Movement Therapies.* Advance online publication. doi:10.1016/j.jbmt.2013.09.011

Lynch, S., & Renstrom, P. (1999). Groin injuries in sport: Treatment strategies. *Sports Medicine, 28*(2), 137–144.

Magee, D. (2007). *Orthopedic physical assessment* (5th ed.). Philadelphia, PA: W. B. Sanders.

Mandelbaum, B., Silvers, H., Watanabe, D., Knarr, J., Thomas, S., Griffin, L., . . . Garrett, W., Jr. (2005). Effectiveness of a neuromuscular and proprioceptive training program in preventing anterior cruciate ligament injuries in female athletes. *American Journal of Sports Medicine, 33*(7), 1003–1010.

Martin, N. M., & Harter, R. A. (1993). Comparison of inversion retraint provided by ankle prophylactic devices before and after exercise. *Journal of Athletic Training, 28*(4), 3245–329.

McDonald, R. (1994). *Taping techniques: Principles and practice.* Oxford, England: Butterworth-Heinemann.

McDonald, R. (2004). *Taping techniques: Principles and practice* (2nd ed.). Oxford, England: Butterworth-Heinemann.

McDonald, R. (2010). *Pocketbook of taping techniques: Principles and practice.* London, England: Churchill Livingstone Elsevier.

Mellion, M., Walsh, W., Madden, C., Putukian, M., & Shelton, G. (2001). *The team physician's handbook* (3rd ed.). Philadelphia, PA: Hanley and Belfus.

Michel, L. M. (1991). Athletic nose guard. Retrieved from http://www.google.com/patents/US5012527?dq=protective+devices+in+athletics

Miller, R., & Dunn, R. (1979). *Athletic training techniques.* Bowling Green, KY: WKU Press.

Myer, G., Ford, K., & Hewett, T. (2004). Rationale and clinical techniques for anterior cruciate ligament injury prevention among female athletes. *Journal of Athletic Training, 39*(4), 352–364.

National Athletic Trainers' Association. (2013, August). Retrieved from http://www.nata.org

National Athletic Trainers' Association. (2005, March). Official statement from the National Athletic Trainers' Association on community-acquired MRSA infection. Retrieved from http://www.nata.org/official-statements

National Center for Safety in Sport. (2012, June). PREPARE sports safety courses. Retrieved from http://www.sportssafety.org

Neumann, D. (2010). *Kinesiology of the musculoskeletal system: Foundations for rehabilitation* (2nd ed.). St. Louis, MO: Mosby Elsevier.

Olmsted, L., Vela, L., & Denegar, C. (2004) Prophylactic ankle taping and bracing: A numbers-needed-to-treat and cost-benefit analysis. *Journal of Athletic Training, 39*(1), 95.

Olmsted-Kramer, L., & Hertel, J. (2004). Preventing recurrent lateral ankle sprains: An evidence-based approach. *Athletic Therapy Today, 9*(6), 19.

Occupational Safety and Health Administration. (2011a). Bloodborne pathogen exposure incidents. Retrieved from https://www.osha.gov/OshDoc/data_BloodborneFacts/bbfact04.pdf

Occupational Safety and Health Administration. (2011b). OSHA's Bloodborne pathogen standard. Retrieved from www.osha.gov/OshDoc/data_BloodborneFacts/bbfact01.pdf

Paris, D. L. (1992). The effects of the swede-o, new cross, and mcdavid ankle braces and adhesive ankle taping on speed, balance, agility, and vertical jump. *Journal of Athletic Training, 27*(3), 253–256.

Perrin, D. (2012). *Athletic taping and bracing* (3rd ed.). Champaign, IL: Human Kinetics.

Pfieffer, R., & Mangus, B. (2011). *Concepts of athletic training* (6th ed.). Boston, MA: Jones and Bartlett.

Porth, C., & Matfin, G. (2009). *Pathophysiology.* Philadelphia, PA: Lippincott Williams & Wilkins.

Prentice, W. (2011). *Principles of athletic training* (14th ed.). New York: McGraw-Hill Higher Education.

Price, S., & Wilson, L. (2002). *Pathophysiology: Clinical concepts of disease processes* (6th ed.). St. Louis, MO: Mosby.

Royal College of Nursing, Society of Orthopaedic and Trauma Nursing. (2012). *A practical guide to casting* (3rd ed.). London, England: BSN Medical.

Ruhi Soylu, A., Irmak, R., & Baltaci, G. (2011). Acute effects of Kinesio Taping on muscular endurance and fatigue by using surface electromyography signals of masseter muscle. *Medicina Sportiva, 15*(1), 13–16.

Starkey, C., Brown, S., & Ryan, J. (2010). *Examination of orthopedic and athletic injuries* (3rd ed.). Philadelphia, PA: F. A. Davis.

Stedman's medical dictionary for the health professions and nursing (7th ed.). (2011). Baltimore, MD: Williams & Wilkins.

Street, S., & Runkle, D. (2000). *Athletic protective equipment: Care, selection, and fitting.* St. Louis, MO: McGraw-Hill Higher Education.

Taber's medical dictionary (22nd ed.). (2012). Philadelphia, PA: F. A. Davis.

Thelen, D., & Stoneman, P. D. (2008). Clinical efficacy of Kinesio® Tape for shoulder pain. *Journal of Orthopaedic & Sports Physical Therapy, 38*(7), 389–395.

Tsai, H.-J., Hung, H.-C., Yang, J.-L., Huang, C.-S., & Tsauo, J.-Y. (2009). Could Kinesio® Tape replace the bandage in decongestive lymphatic therapy. *Supportive Care in Cancer, 17*(11), 1353–1360.

Vithoulka, I., Beneka, A., Malliou, P., Aggelousis, N., Karatsolis, K., & Diamantopoulos, K. (2010). Effects of Kinesio Taping® on quadriceps strength. *Isokinetics and Exercise Science, 18*(1), 1–6.

Wilkerson, G. (2002). Biomechanical and neuromuscular effects of ankle taping and bracing. *Journal of Athletic Training, 37*(4), 436.

Williams, S., Whatman, C., Hume, P. A., & Sheerin, K. (2012). Kinesio taping in treatment and prevention of sports injuries: A meta-analysis of the evidence for its effectiveness. *Sports Medicine, 42*(2), 153–164.

Wright, K., Barker, S., & Whitehill, W. (2007). *Basic athletic training* (5th ed.). Gardner, KS: Cramer Products.

Wright, K., & Deere, R. (1990). Comparison of results concerning the use of ankle taping/strapping and ankle braces. *Applied Research in Coaching and Athletics*, 93–104.

Wright, K., & Hendrix, S. (1989). Perceptions of ankle strapping techniques versus bracing in collegiate basketball. *Sports Medicine Update, 4*(3), 19–20.

Wright, K., & Whitehill, W. (1991). Preparation of the athlete for protective taping/wrapping techniques. *Sports Medicine Update, 6*(1), 26–29.

Wright, K., & Whitehill, W. (1993). How to tape & wrap ankles. *Topics in Sports Medicine, 1*(4), 4–6.

Wright, K., & Whitehill, W. (1996a). *The comprehensive manual of taping and wrapping techniques* (2nd ed.). Gardner, KS: Cramer Products.

Wright, K., & Whitehill, W. (1996b). *Sports medicine taping series* [Video series]. St. Louis: McGraw-Hill Higher Education.

Wright, K., Whitehill, W., & Lewis, M. (2005). Preventive techniques: Taping/wrapping techniques and protective devices (3rd ed.). Gardner, KS: Cramer Products.

Yoshida, A., & Kahanov, L. (2007). The effect of Kinesio Taping on lower trunk range of motions. *Research in Sports Medicine, 15*(2), 103–112.

Appendix C: Websites for Health Care and Sport Industry Professionals

American Academy of Dermatology *www.aad.org*
American Academy of Family Physicians *www.aafp.org*
American Academy of Neurology *www.aan.com*
American Academy of Ophthalmology *www.aao.org*
American Academy of Orthopaedic Surgeons *www.aaos.org*
American Academy of Otolaryngology *www.entnet.org*
American Academy of Pain Management *www.aapainmanage.org*
American Academy of Pediatrics (AAP) *www.aap.org*
American Academy of Podiatric Sports Medicine (AAPSM) *www.aapsm.org*
American Academy of Physical Medicine and Rehabilitation (AAPMR) *www.aapmr.org*
American Chiropractic Association *www.acasc.org*
American College of Foot and Ankle Surgeons *www.acfas.org*
American College of Sports Medicine *www.acsm.org*
American Dental Association *www.ada.org*
American Dietetic Association *www.eatright.org*
American Heart Association *www.americanheart.org*
American Kinesiotherapy Association *www.akta.org*
American Massage Therapy Association *www.amtamassage.org*
American Medical Association *www.ama-assn.org*
American Medical Society for Sport Medicine *www.amssm.org*
American Occupational Therapy Association *www.aota.org*
American Optometric Association *www.aoa.org*
American Orthopaedic Foot and Ankle Society *www.aofas.org*
American Orthopaedic Society for Sports Medicine *www.sportsmed.org*
American Osteopathic Academy of Sport Medicine *www.aoasm.org*
American Osteopathic Association *www.osteopathic.org*
American Physical Therapy Association (APTA) *www.apta.org*
American Physical Therapy Association Sports Physical Therapy Section *www.spts.org*
American Alliance for Health, Physical Education, Recreation, and Dance *www.aahperd.org*
American Association for Physical Activity and Recreation (AAPAR) *www.aapar.org*
America's Health Insurance Plan *www.hiaa.org*
American Red Cross *www.redcross.org*
American Red Cross – Athletic Training Education Competencies *www.redcross.org/athletictrainers*
American Sports Medicine Institute *www.asmi.org*
Athlete Performance Institute *www.athletesperformance.com*

Andrews Institute *www.theandrewsinstitute.com*

Academy for Sports Dentistry (ASD) *www.academyforsportsdentistry.org*

Association for Applied Sport Psychology *www.appliedsportpsych.org*

Association for Sports Medicine in Industry, Business, and Military *www.theindustrialathlete.com*

Association of Sport Performance Centres *http://forumelitesport.org*

Canadian Academy of Sport and Exercise Medicine *www.casem-acmse.org*

Canadian Athletic Therapists Association *www.athletictherapy.org*

Centers for Disease Control and Prevention *www.cdc.gov*

Collegiate Strength and Conditioning Coaches *www.cscca.org*

Collegiate and Professional Sport Dietitians Association (CPSDA) *www.sportrd.org*

International Olympic Committee *www.olympic.org*

International Society for Sports Psychiatry (ISSP) *www.sportspsychiatry.org*

Joint Commission on Sports Medicine and Science *www.jcsportsmedicine.org*

Kinesio Taping Association International *www.kinesiotaping.com/global/association*

Mayo Clinic *www.mayoclinic.org*

National Athletic Trainers' Association *www.nata.org*

National Athletic Trainers' Association Board of Certification *www.bocatc.org*

National Association for Sport and Physical Education *www.aahperd.org/naspe*

National Center for Drug Free Sports *www.drugfreesport.com*

National Center for Sports Safety *www.sportssafety.org*

National Collegiate Athletic Association *www.ncaa.org*

National Federation of State High School Athletic Associations (NFHS) *www.nfhs.org*

NFHS Coach Education *www.nfhslearn.com*

National Interscholastic Athletic Administrators Association *www.niaaa.org*

National Institutes of Health *www.nih.gov*

National Operating Committee on Standards for Athletic Equipment (NOCSEA) *www.nocsae.org*

National Strength and Conditioning Association (NSCA) *www.nsca.com*

National Safety Council *www.nsc.org*

North American Society for Pediatric Exercise Medicine (NASPEM) *www.naspem.org*

Occupational Safety and Health Administration (OSHA) *www.osha.gov*

Sports, Cardiovascular, and Wellness Nutrition (SCAN) *www.scandpg.org*

Sport Information Resource Centre (SIRC) *www.sirc.ca*

Stop Sports Injuries *www.stopsportsinjuries.org*

United States Olympic Committee (USOC) *www.usoc.org*

World Federation of Athletic Training and Therapy *www.wfatt.org*

Appendix D: Websites for Medical Health Care Companies

Medco Sports Medicine *www.medco-athletics.com*

Johnson & Johnson *www.jnj.com*

Kinesio Taping *www.kinesiotaping.com*

Cramer Products, Inc. *www.cramersportsmed.com*

Stromgren Athletics *www.stromgren.com*

Ambra LeRoy Medical *www.ambraleroy.com*

3M *www.3m.com*

DonJoy *www.djoglobal.com*

Amerx Health Care *www.amerigel.com*

Vasyli Medical *www.vasylimedical.com*

Breg *www.breg.com*

Index

Instructions for Online Companion Resource Access

Online companion resources include videos, images, and other resources the authors have provided as supplemental information for the text. These resources are found online and and accessible only by creating an account using the one-time passcode provided at the bottom of this page. For more information about the use of or policies regarding the code for online companion resources, please visit www.sagamorepub.com.

Steps to redeem access code if you DO NOT currently have a Sagamore Account

1. Go to **http://www.sagamorepub.com**

2. Click on the **Create Account** link and fill out the requested information

3. Enter the code provided at the bottom of this page in the **online access code field.**

4. Click on **Create New Account.**

5. Click on **My Materials** tab to access all additional materials provided with your book purchase.

Steps to Redeem Code if you currently DO HAVE a Sagamore Account

1. Go to **http://www.sagamorepub.com**

2. Click on the **Login** link and proceed to login

3. Click on the **Access Codes** tab for your account, enter the code provided at the bottom of this page and click **Submit**.

4. Click on the **My Materials** tab to access all additional materials provided with your book purchase.

Online Materials Access Code

CMT-AQLVME1U7W9O